T0366141

How to
PASS FINALS
Single Best Answers in Medicine

Sanad Esmail
Hasan Haboubi
Jeffrey Stephens

authorHOUSE®

AuthorHouse™ UK
1663 Liberty Drive
Bloomington, IN 47403 USA
www.authorhouse.co.uk
Phone: 0800.197.4150

Published by AuthorHouse   12/23/2014

ISBN: 978-1-4969-9857-6 (sc)
ISBN: 978-1-4969-9858-3 (e)

Contents

Preface

Medical finals are constantly changing, reflecting the dynamic pressures on doctors in training. Whilst the written examinations have evolved with time, the core ethos of it: to act as a benchmark for sound clinical practice, logical diagnostic ability, common sense and most importantly, the development of an applied knowledge of pathophysiology, has remained unchanged.

Whilst this exam has often struck fear into the hearts of students, the authors believe that reinforcing essential learning points through a question/answer format serves as the best way to revise common exam themes.

In 'How to Pass Finals – Single Best Answers in Medicine,' the authors complement a diverse question bank, spanning the vast majority of the medical syllabus, with a thorough set of descriptive answer stems. By doing this, they have created a unified text that can be used as an independent revision resource in its own right, as well as a method of testing a candidate's pre-existing knowledge in preparation for their finals. The questions are presented in a systematic manner according to specialty, which should further aid the revision process.

In producing this book, the authors have utilised their experience as examination question writers. Extensive feedback has also been sought from candidates who have recently sat their medical finals in order to produce a text to better reflect their learning needs. The layout therefore involves a methodical approach with questions set in a single best answer format most modern examinations are undertaken in, and where possible, the cover test has been adhered to, allowing the reader to formulate a diagnosis without needing to read the answer options. Where the cover test is not followed, essential learning points can be derived through exploring the list of possible answer options, thereby expanding the learning opportunities from the relevant questions.

The questions have also been pitched at a greater level of difficulty than that expected of the 'average' final year medical student, ensuring learning potential is optimised. This allows the text to have a dual purpose as a revision tool for medical finals examinations as well improving the readers' likelihood of success by sharpening their knowledge and understanding required for the MRCP written exams.

Finally, and perhaps most uniquely, the book has in parts remained concise with spaces to allow candidates using it to annotate it, thus making it their own personal revision guide. This was a purposeful attempt by the authors to encourage readers to mature their learning process whilst practicing questions.

It must be remembered that there is no substitute for examination practice. Medicine is an art that requires practice. We wish you all the best with your exams and hope that the questions offered in this book will act to complement this practice, polishing your approach to the exam.

"Excellence is an art won by training and habituation. We do not act rightly because we have virtue or excellence, but we rather have those because we have acted rightly. We are what we repeatedly do. Excellence, then, is not an act but a habit."–Aristotle

Sanad Esmail
Hasan Haboubi
Jeffrey Stephens

Author Biographies

Dr Sanad Esmail MBBCh BSc(Hons) MRCP(UK):
Dr Sanad Esmail graduated from the University of Wales College of
Medicine with honours in 2012 after completing a BSc in Neuroscience.
He is currently a Core Medical Trainee in the London Deanery.

Dr Hasan Haboubi MBBS BSc(Hons) MRCP(UK):
Dr Hasan Haboubi graduated from Imperial College London in 2006
and completed his early training in the North West Thames Deanery. He
is currently an Academic Gastroenterology Trainee in the Wales Deanery
and Clinical Lecturer in Swansea University School of Medicine. He has
been heavily involved in teaching at both undergraduate and postgraduate
levels and has run a highly successful finals teaching course since 2006.

Senior Reviewing Author

Professor Jeffrey Stephens BSc MBBS PhD FRCP

Professor Jeffrey W Stephens (BSc, MB BS, PhD, FRCP) qualified in Medicine from St. Mary's Hospital Medical School (Imperial College), London in 1994. He undertook specialist training in Diabetes, Endocrinology and General Internal Medicine throughout Central London. Between 2001-2004 he undertook a PhD in Genetics based at the Centre for Cardiovascular Genetics within the School of Medicine at University College London. He is currently a Clinical Professor of Diabetes at Swansea University and a Consultant Physician in Diabetes, Endocrinology and General Internal Medicine at Morriston Hospital, Swansea. He is actively involved in both teaching and research and continues as a practicing physician in diabetes, endocrinology and general medicine. He has >90 peer reviewed publications. He has extensive teaching experience at medical undergraduate and postgraduate level and also with allied medical specialities. He has previously held positions as Associate Dean for Academic Careers Support within the Wales Deanery, Royal College of Physicians Tutor and Postgraduate Organiser for Morriston Hospital, Swansea.

Endocrinology Questions

1) A 28-year old woman presents to her GP with lethargy, myalgia and a history of recurrent dizzy spells. Her past medical history includes type 1 diabetes.

On examination, she has a tanned appearance, her heart rate is 82/min and regular, blood pressure is 108/72 mmHg. A lying-standing blood pressure reveals a postural drop of 26 mmHg.

Bloods reveal:

Hb	11.2 g/dl (11.5-14.5)	Na⁺ 130mmol/l (135-145)
MCV	86fl (85-100)	K⁺ 5.0 mmol/l (3.5-5)
Platelets	380 x 10⁹/l (150-400)	Creat 116 mmol/l (40-90)
White Cells	8.2 x 10⁹/l (3.5-9)	

What is the most likely diagnosis?

A. Primary adrenocortical insufficiency
B. Secondary adrenocortical insufficiency
C. Cushing's syndrome
D. Haemochromatosis
E. Congenital adrenal hyperplasia

2) A 47-year old lady presents with a lump on the right side of her neck. There have been no symptoms of hyper- or hypothyroidism. She is otherwise fit and well.

She is euthyroid on examination. The right-sided palpable neck lump measures approximately 0.9cm in diameter.

Thyroid stimulating hormone (TSH) levels are 3.2mU/L (0.4-4.4).

What is the most appropriate initial investigation?

A. Final needle aspiration
B. Excisional biopsy
C. CT scan of neck
D. Ultrasound scan of neck
E. Free T3/T4

3) A 74-year old lady is seen in clinic with the following test result:

Adjusted Calcium:	2.80mmol/l (2.2-2.6)
Phosphate:	0.81mmol/l (0.8-1.4)
Parathyroid Hormone (PTH):	4.5pmol/l (0.9-5.4)
Alkaline phosphatase (ALP):	115 U/l (45-105)

She has recently been diagnosed with lung cancer.

What is the most likely diagnosis?

A. Primary hyperparathyroidism
B. Secondary hyperparathyroidism
C. Multiple myeloma
D. Bony metastases
E. Ectopic PTH-related peptide secretion

4) A 35-year old lady presents to her GP because she has had no menstrual periods for the past 6 months despite negative pregnancy tests.
Past medical history includes Grave's disease and vitiligo.
Her GP suspects a diagnosis of premature ovarian failure.

Which of the following investigation findings would be most consistent with this?

A. Elevated oestradiol
B. Low LH
C. Low GnRH
D. Elevated testosterone
E. Elevated FSH

5) A 37-year old lady presents to the clinic with palpitations and heat intolerance. On examination she appears irritable, her BMI is 20, blood pressure is 128/78 mmHg and her pulse is 98 irregularly irregular.
TSH is suppressed at <0.05.

Which of the following features would you most likely expect given this clinical picture?

A. Increased libido
B. Menorrhagia
C. Coarse resting tremor
D. Diarrhoea
E. Dry skin

6) A 52-year old man with Type 2 Diabetes Mellitus is started on Liraglutide (Victoza).

Which of the following regarding its mechanism of action is INCORRECT?

A. Activates GLP-1 receptors
B. Inhibits gastric emptying
C. Stimulates insulin release
D. Inhibits glucagon output
E. Associated with weight gain

7) A 43-year old woman presents with polydipsia and polyuria.

Which of the following would confirm a diagnosis of diabetes mellitus? (Normal blood glucose 4.4-6.1 mmol/l)

A. A 2 hour OGTT glucose level of 10.8 mmol/l
B. A random blood glucose level of 9.6 mmol/l
C. A fasting blood glucose of 6.8 mmol/l
D. Urine dipstick with glucose +++
E. HbA1c of 58 mmol/mol (20-41)

8) A 48-year old asymptomatic female with a strong family history of type 2 diabetes mellitus is shown to have a fasting plasma glucose of 6.3 mmol/l (4.4-6.1).

Which of the following is correct regarding the next most appropriate plan?

A. Repeat fasting glucose after 4 weeks
B. Repeat fasting glucose after 8 weeks
C. Perform an oral glucose tolerance test (OGTT)
D. Commence treatment for type 2 diabetes
E. No further investigation necessary

9) Which of the following is NOT associated with acromegaly?

A. Cardiomyopathy
B. Carpal tunnel syndrome
C. Hypertension
D. Anhydrosis
E. Colorectal cancer

10) A 43-year old gentleman is reviewed in clinic after noticing gradual, progressive coarsening of his facial appearance. He states his shoes no longer fit him and he's unable to wear his wedding ring as it is now too tight.

On examination, there is prognathism and prominent supra-orbital ridges.

Which of the following is the most appropriate initial screening test?

A. Insulin tolerance test
B. Growth hormone levels
C. IGF-1 levels
D. Oral glucose tolerance test
E. MRI of pituitary gland

11) A 43-year old male presents with lethargy, decreased libido and erectile dysfunction. Serum prolactin is measured at 800 U/L (< 450U/l in men is normal). His medication list includes Metoclopramide, Phenytoin, Metformin, Ramipril and Amiodarone.

   Which of the following drugs is most likely to cause this clinical presentation?

   A. Metoclopramide
   B. Phenytoin
   C. Metformin
   D. Ramipril
   E. Amiodarone

12) A 32-year old female presents with weight gain and intermittent episodes of intense sweating and palpitations.

   What is the most appropriate diagnostic investigation?

   A. 24 hour urinary catecholamines
   B. 24 hour urinary 5-hydroxyindoleacetic acid (5-HIAA)
   C. MRI adrenals
   D. Thyroid function tests
   E. Prolonged (72 hour) supervised fast

13) A patient is seen in the pre-operative assessment clinic. He is due to undergo a laparoscopic adrenalectomy for a phaeochromocytoma but remains hypertensive with a blood pressure of 160/102 mmHg.

   Which of the following anti-hypertensives should be initiated first?

   A. Atenolol
   B. Phenoxybenzamine
   C. Propanolol
   D. Amlodipine
   E. Methyldopa

14) Which of the following hormones exerts its physiological effects through the tyrosine receptor kinase signalling system?

A. TRH
B. TSH
C. Oestradiol
D. Glucagon
E. Insulin

15) A 36-year old male presents with headache and paroxysmal episodes of palpitations, sweating and flushing. He is on ramipril, amlodipine and bendroflumethiazide for hypertension. Past medical history includes previous thyroidectomy for thyroid cancer.

On examination, he has a normal body habitus, heart rate is 78/min regular and blood pressure is 164/94 mmHg.

What is the most likely diagnosis?

A. Multiple Endocrine Neoplasia type 1
B. Multiple Endocrine Neoplasia type 2a
C. Multiple Endocrine Neoplasia type 2b
D. Autoimmune polyendocrine syndrome type 1
E. Autommune polyendocrine syndrome type 2

16) A 38-year old female presents with a 2-month history of weight loss despite increased appetite and heat intolerance.

On examination, she appears anxious and has a fine resting tremor. A diffuse goitre is palpable.

Thyroid function tests reveal:

Free T3   11.1 pmol/l (4-8.3)

Free T4   42 pmol/l (10-24)

TSH   4.2 mU/l (0.4-4.5)

What is the most appropriate investigation?

A. Anti-TSH receptor antibodies
B. Anti-TPO antibodies
C. Final needle aspiration of thyroid
D. MRI pituitary
E. Radio-iodine uptake scan of thyroid

17) Which of the following thyroid profiles is most consistent with subclinical hypothyroidism?

(Normal values: free T3 (4-8.3pmol/l), free T4 (10-24pmol/l), TSH (0.4-4.5mU/l))

A. Free T3: 3.2, Free T4: 8, TSH: 4.1
B. Free T3: 2.1, Free T4: 5.4, TSH: 14.2
C. Free T3: 4.6, Free T4: 18.3, TSH: 9.6
D. Free T3: 6.3, Free T4: 12.2, TSH: 0.1
E. Free T3: 10.8, Free T4: 26.1, TSH: 0.2

18) A 48-year old male attends clinic for review. Past medical history includes gallstones, hypertension and a 10-year history of type II diabetes for which she is on metformin 500mg three times daily. She drinks 16 units of alcohol per week.

On examination, she is obese with a BMI of 31 kg/m². Liver function tests reveal:

Bilirubin	10 μmol/l (1-20)
Alkaline Phosphatase (ALP)	122 U/L (25-110)
Alanine Transaminase (ALT)	120 U/L (5-45)
Aspartate Transaminase (AST)	84 U/L (5-45 U/L)
Gamma-glutamyl transpepdidase (γ-GT)	60 U/L (6-42)
Albumin	32 g/l (33-49)
Glycated Haemoglobin (HbA1C)	68 mmol/mol (20-41)

An ultrasound scan of the abdomen shows bright areas of echogenicity in the liver and multiple calculi in the gallbladder.

What is the most likely diagnosis?

A. Non-alcoholic steatohepatitis
B. Autoimmune hepatitis
C. Drug-induced hepatitis
D. Alcohol-related liver disease
E. Gallstone-related liver disease

19) A serum prolactin level from a 32-year-old lady is shown to be elevated at 750 u/L (<600 normal in women).

Which of the following is the most likely diagnosis?

A. Primary hypothyroidism
B. Primary hyperthyroidism
C. Microprolactinoma
D. Macroprolactinoma
E. Hyperprolactinaemia secondary to cabergoline therapy

20) You are presented with the following Urea and Electrolyte results:

Na$^+$	128 mmol/l
K$^+$	3.1 mmol/l
Urea	6.5 mmol/l
Creat	68micromol/l
Adj Ca^{2+}	2.74 mmol/l

Which diuretic is most likely to cause this type of biochemical profile?

A. Furosemide
B. Spironolactone
C. Amiloride
D. Bendroflumethiazide
E. Bumetanide

21) You have been asked to review a patient by the chest team. She is an 88-year-old lady who was initially managed as community acquired pneumonia. On admission 2 days ago, she had a serum sodium of 120mmol/l (normal range 135-145). However, looking through her history you note that only 3 weeks previously her serum sodium was within the normal range.

Her past medical history includes hypothyroidism, hypertension and cataracts.

She takes Levothyroxine 100 micrograms, Furosemide 40mg, Amlodipine 10mg and Ramipril 5mg, each once daily.

The patient is euvolaemic on examination.

Investigations reveal:

Short synacthen test:	Normal	
TSH:	4.0	(0.4-4.5)
Serum Osmolality:	258	(285-295 mOsm/kg)
Urine Osmolality:	300	(50-1400 mOsm/kg)
Urine sodium:	> 40	(>40mmol/l)
Serum Na$^+$	116	(135-145mmol/l)

Which of the following is the first most appropriate treatment option?

A. Increase the levothyroxine to 125 micrograms/day
B. Trial of demeclocycline 300mg twice daily
C. Fluid restrict 800 ml/day
D. Infusion of hypertonic saline
E. Stop furosemide and ramipril

22) A 48-year old publican is reviewed in the diabetes clinic. He has type 2 diabetes diagnosed 1 year ago, which is diet-controlled. He suffers from chronic kidney disease and has a history of heart failure.

On examination, he is overweight with a BMI of 28 kg/m^2.

Bloods reveal:

Na$^+$	135mmol/l (135-145)
K$^+$	4.8mmol/l (3.5-5)
Urea	4.6 mmol/l (2-8)
Creat	152micromol/l (40-90)
HbA1c	59 mmol/mol (20-41)

Which of the following is the next most appropriate treatment?

A. Metformin
B. Gliclazide
C. Glibenclamide
D. Pioglitazone
E. Insulin

23) Which of the following correctly describes the mechanism of action of metformin?

A. Inhibits hepatic gluconeogenesis
B. Stimulates insulin secretion
C. Activates PPAR-alpha receptors
D. Activates PPAR-gamma receptors
E. Inhibits dipeptidyl peptidase IV (DPP-IV) enzymes

24) You review the blood results of a 29-year old female patient known to suffer from chronic alcoholism. She originally presented 3 days previously with alcohol withdrawal and was initially treated with diazepam as per CIWA and intravenous pabrinex. Bloods are as follows:

Na$^+$	130 mmol/l (135-145)
K$^+$	2.8 mmol/l (3.5-5.3)
Urea	3.6 mmol/l (2.5-7.5)
Creat	76 micromol/l (40-90)

Despite two consecutive bags of 0.9% normal saline with 40 mmol/l KCL, she remains hypokalaemic (K$^+$ still 2.8mmol/l).

Which of the following minerals should be measured?

A. Calcium
B. Magnesium
C. Zinc
D. Phosphate
E. Copper

25) You review the blood results of a critically unwell patient:

Na$^+$	150 mmol/l (135-145)
K$^+$	5.0 mmol/l (3.5-5.3)
Urea	15.0 mmol/l (2.5-7.5)
Creat	190 micromol/l (40-90)
Glucose	45 mmol/l (4.4-6.1)
Ketones	0.8 mmol/l (<0.6)

What is the plasma osmolality (mOsm/kg)?

A. 315
B. 330
C. 345
D. 360
E. 380

26) An 18-year old male student with type 1 diabetes presents to the emergency department with a 4-day history of polydipsia, polyuria and cough productive of green sputum. On examination, there is bronchial breathing in the left base, he is pyrexial at 38.4 degrees, heart rate is 118/min regular and blood pressure is 122/76 mmHg.

Investigations reveal:

Haemoglobin	13.6 g/dl (11.5-14)
White Cell Count	18.6 x 10^9/l (3.5-9)
Neutrophils	16.4 x 10^9/l (1.2-7.7)
Venous lactate	2.6 mmol/l (1-2)
Bicarbonate	12.0 mmol/l (24-30)
Capillary ketones	6 mmol/l (<0.6)
Plasma glucose	28 mmol/l (4.4-6.1)

Chest X-ray: consolidation of the left lower zone

Which of the following is the most important immediate management?

A. Variable rate sliding scale insulin infusion
B. Fixed rate insulin infusion
C. Intravenous antibiotics
D. Blood cultures
E. Intravenous fluid resuscitation

27) A 73-year old male is brought into the medical assessment unit with severe lethargy and feeling generally unwell.

Past medical history includes ischaemic heart disease and type II diabetes controlled with metformin and gliclazide. On examination, he weighs 70 kg and is clinically very dry.

Bloods reveal:

Na^+	155 mmol/l (135-145)
K^+	4.0 mmol/l (3.5-5)
Urea	15.0 mmol/l (2.5-7.5)
Creat	180 micromol/l (40-89)
Glucose	40 mmol/l (4.4-6.1)
Capillary ketones	0.6 mmol/l (<0.6)

Which of the following statements regarding this condition is FALSE?

A. The most likely diagnosis is Hyperosmolar Hyperglycaemic state
B. Plasma osmolality is 373 mOsm/kg
C. Plasma osmolality should be corrected at a rate of 10-14 mOsm/kg/hour
D. Fluid deficit is around 7-15 litres
E. When insulin is commenced, it should be at a fixed rate of 3.5 units/hour

28) A 35-year old patient is clerked in the medical assessment unit. A diagnosis of Addison's disease is suspected.

Which of the following would be the most useful investigation?

A. Short synacthen test
B. Random serum cortisol
C. Dexamethasone suppression test
D. Serum ACE
E. Insulin tolerance test

29) A 20-year old 70kg patient with known type 1 diabetes is treated for diabetic ketoacidosis (DKA).

What is the likely volume of fluid deficit?

A. 1-2 litres
B. 2-3 litres
C. 4-5 litres
D. 6-8 litres
E. 9-11 litres

30) A mother brings her 1-month-old child to the endocrine clinic for review. She is concerned as her daughter has been suffering from repeated bouts of vomiting and is failing to gain weight.

On examination, there is reduced skin turgor, sunken eyes and ambiguous genitalia.

Investigations reveal hyperkalaemia, hyponatraemia and hyper-reninaemia.

Which enzyme is most likely to be deficient?

A. 3-beta-hydroxysteroid dehydrogenase
B. 5-alpha reductase
C. 11-beta hydroxylase
D. 18-hydroxylase
E. 21-alpha hydroxylase

31) Which part of the adrenal gland is cortisol synthesised?

A. Adrenal capsule
B. Adrenal medulla
C. Zona glomerulosa
D. Zona fasciculata
E. Zona reticularis

32) A 36-year old male is reviewed in clinic. He presents with a 3-month history of progressive weight gain and truncal obesity.

On examination, there is supraclavicular fullness and a dorsocervical fat pad.

Past medical history includes alcoholism, hypertension and depression.

Blood pressure is 168/92 mmHg, heart rate is 72/min regular and temperature is 36.8 degrees.

Investigations reveal:

24-hour urinary free cortisol: 460 nmol (normal < 280 nmol)
Low dose dexamethasone suppression test: negative

What is the most likely diagnosis?

A. Pseudo-Cushing's syndrome
B. Cushing's syndrome
C. Cushing's disease
D. Nelson's syndrome
E. Ectopic ACTH syndrome

33) Which of the following is the gold-standard investigation for confirming an ACTH-secreting pituitary adenoma?

A. 24-houry urinary free cortisol
B. Low dose dexamethasone suppression test
C. High dose dexamethasone suppression test
D. Pituitary MRI
E. Bilateral inferior petrosal sinus sampling

34) A male type II diabetic patient is reviewed in clinic.

He is on metformin, gliclazide and 20 units of insulin glargine taken at night.

Despite these measures, his morning fasting plasma glucose is consistently 12-15 mmol/l (4-5.9mmol/l pre-prandial, <7.8mmol/l post-prandial) and his HbA1c is 58 mmol/mol (20-41mmol/l).

His blood sugars before lunch and dinner are within the normal range.

What is the next most appropriate management option?

A. Stop metformin and gliclazide and commence basal bolus regimen
B. Start basal bolus regimen and increase insulin glargine by 2-4 units
C. Increase insulin glargine by 2-4 units only
D. Add a GLP-1 analogue
E. Measure plasma glucose at 3-5am over several nights and adjust insulin glargine accordingly

35) A 48-year old lady is referred to the endocrine clinic with secondary amenorrhoea and infertility. On examination, she is obese with a BMI of 34 kg/m², has evidence of hirsutism and acne.

Bloods during the luteal phase reveal:

Hb	13.6g/dl (11.4-14)
LH	21 u/L (3-16)
FSH	10 u/L (1-11)
Testosterone	8 nmol/l (0.4-2.4)

24-hour urinary free cortisol: 340 nmol (< 280)

Transvaginal ultrasound: multiple loculated ovarian cysts

What is the most likely diagnosis?

A. Stein-Leventhal syndrome
B. Late-onset congenital adrenal hyperplasia
C. Cushing's syndrome
D. Simple obesity
E. Androgen-secreting tumour

36) A 17-year old female presents with primary amenorrhoea.

Past medical history includes bilateral inguinal hernia repair as a child. Fluorescence in situ hybridisation reveals an XY karyotype.

What is the most likely diagnosis?

A. Androgen insensitivity syndrome
B. Klinefelter's syndrome
C. Turner's syndrome
D. Kallmann syndrome
E. Noonan's syndrome

37) A 22-year old male presents with polydipsia, polyuria and nocturia.

Which of the following does NOT produce this clinical presentation?

A. Hyperglycaemia
B. Lithium therapy
C. Hypocalcaemia
D. Hypokalaemia
E. Cranial diabetes inspidus

38) A patient with known Addison's disease takes 20mg of hydrocortisone in the morning and 10mg in the evening.

What total daily dose of prednisolone does this translate to?

A. 2.5mg
B. 5mg
C. 7.5mg
D. 10mg
E. 12.5mg

39) A 28-year old female who is 1-day post-thyroidectomy complains of perioral tingling and numbness.
Chvostek's sign is positive.

What is the most likely cause for this abnormality?

A. Hypocalcaemia
B. Hypercalcaemia
C. Hyperphosphataemia
D. Hypophosphataemia
E. Nerve Injury

40) Which of the following statements regarding osteoporosis and its management is FALSE?

A. A diagnosis of osteoporosis is made with a T score < -2.5
B. Raloxifene works as an oestrogen receptor agonist
C. Thyrotoxicosis is a recognised cause of secondary osteoporosis
D. Bisphosphonates inhibits osteoclast-mediated bone resorption
E. Osteoporosis more frequently affects women than men

Endocrinology Answers

1) A: Primary adrenocortical insufficiency

The diagnosis is Addison's disease, also known as primary adrenocortical insufficiency. The most common cause in developed countries is autoimmune adrenalitis (>90% of causes in the UK), whilst in the developing world it's tuberculous adrenalitis (occurring in around 5% of active tuberculosis).

Addison's disease is a rare condition with an incidence of only 4.7-6.2 per million in white populations. It commonly presents with vague symptoms including fatigue, lethargy, anorexia, weight loss, nausea, vomiting, presyncope/syncope, abdominal pain (occasionally mimicking an acute abdomen), arthralgia and myalgia. Thus, making a diagnosis requires a high index of suspicion.

Addison's disease is characterised by a lack of cortisol and aldosterone synthesis. Cortisol helps to maintain the sensitivity of the vasculature to adrenaline and noradrenaline, thus permitting vasoconstriction. Aldosterone drives salt and water retention, whilst stimulating potassium excretion from the kidneys; thus aldosterone deficiency is responsible for the combination of hyponatraemia and hyperkalaemia. Low levels of cortisol and aldosterone collectively explain the tendency to postural hypotension (systolic drop of >20mmHg from lying to standing) and recurrent episodes of presyncope or syncope.

Cortisol production is driven by activity in the hypothalamic-pituitary axis. Specifically, corticotrophin-releasing hormone (CRH) from the hypothalamus stimulates adrenocorticotrophic hormone (ACTH) secretion from the anterior pituitary, which subsequently stimulates cortisol synthesis from the adrenal cortex. In Addison's disease, deficient cortisol induces elevations in CRH and ACTH owing to blunted negative feedback effects. The high ACTH is associated with high melanocyte-stimulating hormone (MSH) as both molecules are derived from the same precursor. Melanocyte stimulation consequently explains the skin hyperpigmentation and tanned appearance in Addison's disease. The tanned appearance and mineralocorticoid deficiency does not occur in secondary adrenocortical insufficiency.

Arit W and Allolio B. Adrenal insufficiency. Lancet. 2003;361: 1881-93

2) D: Ultrasound scan of neck

An ultrasound scan is often the investigation of choice in patients presenting with neck lumps who are clinically euthyroid. Ultrasound will reveal the consistency of the lump (i.e. cystic or solid), which will guide further investigation; fine needle aspiration cytology for cystic lumps or excisional biopsy for solid lumps.

3) A: Primary hyperparathyroidism

Although multiple myeloma, bony metastases and ectopic PTH-related peptide secretion can cause hypercalcaemia, the PTH would be suppressed to below the normal value. In this case, the PTH is inappropriately normal and its lack of suppression makes a diagnosis of primary hyperparathyroidism most likely.

4) E: Elevated FSH

Given this patient's history of Grave's disease and vitiligo, she is at increased risk of other autoimmune-mediated conditions, including premature (or primary) ovarian failure. The premature shutdown of oestrogen production liberates the gonadotrophins from feedback inhibition, thus resulting in elevated levels of FSH and LH.

Nippita TA and Baber RJ. Premature ovarian failure: a review. Climacteric. 2007;10: 11-22

5) D: Diarrhoea

This patient presents with hyperthyroidism. Classical symptoms include weight loss despite increased appetite, irritability, heat intolerance, excessive sweating, palpitations, increased bowel frequency and in women, oligomenorrhoea. Signs include tachycardia, atrial fibrillation, warm moist skin, fine resting tremor and in the case of Graves disease, diffuse painless goiter, ophthalmopathy (causing lid lag and exophthalmos) and rarely pretibial myxedema.

Hyperthyroidism can be divided into primary and secondary forms. Primary hyperthyroidism is when there is autonomous hypersecretion of thyroxine from the thyroid. This is most commonly due to Graves disease, an autoimmune process characterised by the production of stimulatory anti-TSH receptor autoantibodies. Other less frequent causes of primary hyperthyroidism include toxic multinodular goitre and toxic adenomas. Secondary hyperthyroidism, which is far less common, is when thyrotoxicosis occurs secondary to pathology in another organ, resulting in excess thyroid stimulation. This can occur due to a TSH-secreting pituitary adenoma or excessive TRH release from the hypothalamus for example. As the TSH is suppressed in this question, the cause is primary hyperthyroidism.

Nygaard B. Hyperthyroidism. American Family Physician. 2007;76: 1014-16.

6) E: Associated with weight gain

Liraglutide (trade name Victoza) is a glucagon-like peptide-1 (GLP-1) analogue that works via the incretin effect. Like the endogenous incretins (GLP-1 and gastric inhibitory peptide (GIP)), liraglutide and other GLP-1 analogues including exenatide, function to stimulate insulin release, inhibit glucagon output, inhibit gastric emptying and are associated with the prevention of weight gain and possibly weight loss. According to NICE recommendations, the GLP-1 analogues can be used as an adjunct in the treatment of type II diabetes once glycaemic control is deemed inadequate with metformin and a sulphonylurea providing certain criteria are fulfilled (e.g. if BMI >35 or, if BMI<35 and insulin therapy is unacceptable for occupational reasons or weight loss would benefit other significant obesity-related comorbidities).

The DPP-4 inhibitors (e.g. saxagliptin, sitagliptin and vildagliptin) work by inhibiting the enzyme dipeptidyl peptidase-4 (DPP-4), which normally breaks down GLP-1. Thus, by raising the levels of endogenous GLP-1, the DPP-4 inhibitors create similar physiological effects to the GLP-1 analogues.

British Medical Association and the Royal Pharmaceutical Society of Great Britain. British National Formulary. 61st edition. UK: BMJ Publishing Group. 2011.

National Institute for Health and Clinical Excellence. 2010. Liraglutide for the treatment of type 2 diabetes mellitus. CG 203. London: National Institute for Health and Clinical Excellence.

7) **E: HbA1c of 58 mmol/mol**

According to guidelines from the World Health Organisation (WHO), a diagnosis of diabetes can be made if there are corresponding symptoms (e.g. polydipsia, polyuria or unexplained weight loss) and:

a)   Fasting plasma glucose more than 7 mmol/l or
b)   Random plasma glucose more than 11.1 mmol/l or
c)   Plasma glucose of more than 11.1 mmol/l 2 hours after a glucose load of 75g solution consumed within 5 minutes (the 2 hour Oral Glucose Tolerance Test (OGTT)).

If there are no symptoms, then a positive fasting, random or OGTT on 2 separate occasions confirms the diagnosis.

Glycated haemoglobin (HbA1C) is often used as an objective measure of average blood glucose control during the preceding 8 to 12 weeks, correlating with the average lifespan of an erythrocyte. More recently, recommendations from WHO have suggested that a diagnosis of diabetes can be made if the HbA1C is more than 48 mmol/mol (6.5%). Again, if there are no symptoms, the HbA1C should be repeated on 2 separate occasions. However, there are limitations to using the HbA1C in this way (e.g. cannot be used to diagnose patients who are acutely ill, are very young, pregnant etc).

WHO. Use of glycated haemoglobin (HbA1c) in the diagnosis of diabetes mellitus. 2011.

Farmer A. Use of HbA1C in the diagnosis of diabetes. British Medical Journal. 2012;345: e7293

8) **C: Perform an oral glucose tolerance test (OGTT)**

A fasting glucose of 6.1-6.9 mmol/l is suggestive of impaired fasting glycaemia. Such patients are at high risk of developing diabetes and according to WHO recommendations, require further investigation with an OGTT.

A 2-hour plasma glucose in an OGTT of 7.8-11.1 mmol/l is suggestive of impaired glucose tolerance. Again, these patients are at increased risk of developing type 2 diabetes.

9) **D: Anhydrosis**

Acromegaly is typically associated with increased sweating and not anhydrosis. All other options are recognised clinical features of acromegaly. By stimulating the formation and growth of adenomatous polyps, which can gain malignant potential, acromegaly is known to increase the risk of colorectal cancer and patients should be offered screening colonoscopy.

10) **C: IGF-1 levels**

The diagnosis is acromegaly. It is characterised by growth hormone (GH) hypersecretion, 95% of which occur secondary to a pituitary adenoma (the remainder being caused by ectopic production of GH and GH-releasing hormone (GHRH).

GH is secreted in a pulsatile manner by the anterior pituitary, explaining why measuring a random GH level provides very little useful information. GH release is stimulated by GHRH and inhibited by somatostatin, the latter 2 hormones being produced by the hypothalamus and reaching the anterior pituitary via the hypothalamic-hypophyseal portal venous system.

GH stimulates IGF-1, which is predominantly produced by the liver. IGF-1 levels provide a more reliable indicator of average GH levels and therefore provide a useful screening measure. If IGF-1 is raised, an oral glucose tolerance test (OGTT) can subsequently be performed. Failure of GH suppression to less than 1 microgram/L after consumption of 75g of glucose represents a positive test result and is virtually diagnostic of acromegaly.

After a positive OGTT, an MRI of the pituitary should subsequently be carried out in order to identify a potential pituitary adenoma. Treatment of choice is most often transphenoidal surgery unless patient preference dictates otherwise or the tumour is unlikely to be fully resected due to its size or site of invasion (e.g. if the cavernous sinuses are involved). Conservative management includes somatostatin analogues, namely octreotide and lanreotide.

Rarely, in the case of a normal pituitary, further investigations should be pursued, including a CT chest and abdomen to exclude any ectopic GH or GHRH-releasing tumours.

Melmed S. Acromegaly. The New England Journal of Medicine. 2006;355:2558-73

11) A: Metoclopramide

Hyperprolactinaemia frequently presents with decreased libido and erectile dysfunction in men, and as galactorrhoea, oligo- or amenorrhoea and infertility in women. Patients also commonly present with lethargy and, in the case of pituitary tumours, headaches and visual field defects.

Prolactin secretion from the anterior pituitary lactotrophs is normally under inhibitory control by dopamine, which is secreted by the hypothalamic neurons into the hypophyseal portal venous system. Thus, drugs that antagonize the effects of dopamine can dampen this inhibitory control and raise prolactin levels. Metoclopramide, being a dopamine receptor antagonist, is thus most likely, from the list of possible options, to cause hyperprolactinaemia. Other drugs strongly implicated in raising prolactin levels include antipsychotics, antidepressants, opiates, H2-receptor antagonists amongst others.

La Torre D and Falomi A. Pharmacological causes of hyperprolactinemia. Journal of Therapeutics and Clinical Risk Management. 2007;3: 929-51

12) E: Prolonged (72 hour) supervised fast

Although paroxysms of sweating and palpitations are characteristics of phaeochromocytoma, weight gain does not typically feature, explaining why options a) and c) are incorrect.

Although intense sweating and palpitations are symptoms of thyrotoxicosis, weight gain is associated with hypothyroidism. This makes a pathology of the thyroid unlikely, thereby explaining why option d) is incorrect.

The diagnosis is an insulinoma, whereby excessive levels of endogenous insulin cause weight gain and intermittent hypoglycaemic episodes, which explain the periods of intense sweating and palpitations. The diagnosis is supported by a supervised prolonged fast typically lasting up to 72 hours. If the patient develops symptoms, blood is taken for plasma glucose, insulin and c-peptide. Abnormally low levels of glucose alongside raised (or inappropriately 'normal') levels of insulin and c-peptide confirm the diagnosis. In cases of exogenous insulin overdoses, plasma insulin will be high, but this will not be accompanied by raised c-peptide, as c-peptide is only present in endogenous insulin.

13) B: Phenoxybenzamine

Phaeochromocytomas are catecholamine-secreting tumours of the chromaffin cells arising from the adrenal medulla or extra-adrenal paraganglia in approximately 85% and 15% of cases, respectively. It is a rare cause of hypertension affecting 0.1-0.6% of the general population. Patients can present with paroxysms of hypertensive episodes, headaches, palpitations, sweats and feelings of intense panic. Useful investigations include 24-hour urine collections for urinary catecholamines, vanillylmandelic acid and metanephrines, which would all be significantly raised in phaeochromocytoma patients. Imaging the adrenal glands may reveal tumours amenable to surgery.

When pre-operatively managing hypertension in phaechromocytoma patients, it is essential to commence alpha-blockade (i.e.

phenoxybenzamine) prior to beta-blockade. Blocking beta receptors first can potentially exacerbate hypertension by inducing peripheral vasoconstriction.

Lenders JW, Eisenhofer G, Mannelli M and Pacak K. Pheochromocytoma. Lancet. 2005; 366:665-75

14) E: Insulin

The following shows examples of different intracellular signalling cascades and the corresponding hormones:

a) Tyrosine receptor kinase – insulin
b) cAMP messenger system – TSH, adrenaline, LH, FSH, PTH, glucagon
c) cGMP messenger system – nitric oxide and atrial natriuretic peptide (ANP)
d) Phosphoinositide signalling cascade – TRH, ADH
e) Steroid receptor signalling – oestradiol, testosterone, cortisol, progesterone

15) B: Multiple Endocrine Neoplasia type 2a

This patient presents with clinical features of pheochromocytoma, which in a small proportion of patients is inherited as part of multiple endocrine neoplasia (MEN) type 2, a rare familial cancer syndrome.

Patients with MEN type 1 develop parathyroid adenomas, pituitary adenomas and pancreatic neuroendocrine tumours (e.g. insulinomas, gastrinomas, VIPomas etc).

Patients with MEN type 2 develop parathyroid hyperplasia (less frequently adenoma), medullary thyroid cancer and pheochromocytoma, although as in MEN type 1, not all features are necessarily present simultaneously. MEN type 2 can be further subdivided into type 2a and type 2b. Type 2b patients classically have a tall and thin Marfanoid-like appearance, and frequently develop mucosal neuromas. These are absent in MEN 2a.

MEN syndromes are inherited in an autosomal dominant pattern of inheritance.

In this example, the thyroidectomy was probably because of medullary thyroid cancer.

The autoimmune polyglandular syndromes are associated with endocrine organ deficiency rather than over-activity. Type 1 refers to a combination of hypoparathyroidism and Addisons disease, usually in association with candidiasis. Type 2 (Schmidt's) encompasses features of Addison's disease, hypothyroidism and type 1 diabetes mellitus.

Lakhani VT, You N and Wells SA. The Multiple Endocrine Neoplasia Syndromes. Annual Review of Medicine. 2007;58: 253-65.

16) D: MRI pituitary

Thyroxine normally exerts a negative feedback effect on its release from the thyroid by inhibiting TSH secretion from the anterior pituitary. Failure of TSH suppression in the presence of high levels of free T3 and T4 suggests secondary hyperthyroidism. Imaging of the pituitary gland to identify the presence of a TSH-secreting pituitary tumour would therefore be the most appropriate investigation. If TSH levels were suppressed, then anti-TSH receptor antibody levels would be most appropriate in order to exclude or confirm a diagnosis of Grave's disease, the most common cause of primary hyperthyroidism.

Nygaard B. Hyperthyroidism. American Family Physician. 2007;76: 1014-16.

17) C: Free T3: 4.6, Free T4: 18.3, TSH: 9.6

Options A) and E) are consistent with primary hypothyroidism and hyperthyroidism, respectively. Low levels of free T3, T4 and TSH represent secondary hypothyroidism or can be compatible with sick euthyroid syndrome, whereas high levels of all these hormones represent secondary hyperthyroidism.

Normal free T3 and T4 levels combined with elevated TSH is subclinical hypothyroidism (option C), whereas normal free T3 and T4 along with suppressed TSH is consistent with subclinical hyperthyroidism (option D).

Dayan CM. Interpretation of thyroid function tests. Lancet. 2001;357: 619-24

18) A: Non-alcoholic steatohepatitis

Non-alcoholic steatohepatitis (NASH) is an increasingly common cause of liver inflammation and is strongly associated with insulin resistance, obesity and hyperlipidaemia. This patient's long-history of diabetes, which is poorly controlled given an HbA1C of 68 (target is 48 mmol/mol), and obesity places him at high risk of NASH. The brightly echogenic appearance of the liver provides evidence of fatty infiltration. The hepatitic pattern of liver function test results is further supportive of NASH. Gallstone-related liver disease would produce a far greater rise in ALP and gamma GT.

In Non Alcoholic Fatty Liver Disease, the AST:ALT ratio is usually <1 (compared to Alcoholic Liver Disease where the ratio is usually >2).

19) A: Primary hypothyroidism

Micro and macroprolactinomas tend to produce far greater levels of prolactin. Microprolactinomas produce prolactin levels of up to 5000u/L, whereas macroprolactinomas produce greater elevations of up to 10,000 u/L or more. Hyperthyroidism and cabergoline therapy are not associated with raised prolactin levels; in fact, being a dopamine agonist, cabergoline is used in the treatment of hyperprolactinaemia.

Primary hypothyroidism can produce mild elevations of prolactin because the high TRH levels resulting from a reduced negative feedback effect on the hypothalamus can stimulate the anterior pituitary and raise prolactin secretion.

Clinical symptoms of hypothyroidism include fatigue, lethargy, weight gain, cognitive slowing and cold intolerance. Signs include dry skin, thinning of the hair, slow-relaxing tendon reflexes and bradycardia.

Melmed S, Casanueva FF, Hoffman AR et al. Diagnosis and Treatment of Hyperprolactinemia: An Endocrine Society Clinical Practise Guideline.

20) D: Bendroflumethiazide

The combination of hyponatraemia, hypokalaemia and hypercalcaemia can be caused by thiazide diuretic. Furosemide and bumetanide are both loop diuretics, which although often produce hyponatraemia and hypokalaemia, typically cause hypocalcaemia instead of a raised calcium. Loop diuretics work by inhibiting the sodium, potassium, chloride co-transporter in the thick ascending limb of the loop of henle. Spironolactone and amiloride are potassium-sparing diuretics and so tend not to produce hypokalaemia.

Thiazides can cause hypercalcaemia because by inhibiting the sodium-chloride co-transporter in the distal convoluted tubule apical membranes, they raise the concentration gradient of sodium ions and increase the activity of sodium-calcium antiporters on the basolateral membranes. This leads to an increased absorption of calcium ions from the kidneys into the systemic circulation.

Brater DC. Diuretic Therapy. The New England Journal of Medicine. 1998; 339: 387-95.

21) E: Stop furosemide and ramipril

The cause of hyponatraemia in this patient is multifactorial being a combination of drug-induced hyponatraemia and syndrome of inappropriate ADH release (SIADH). SIADH is a diagnosis of exclusion and requires the following criteria to be met:

a) Hyponatraemia
b) Inappropriately concentrated urine (> 100mOsm/kg, but is often higher than serum osmolality)
c) Urine sodium > 40mmol/l
d) Normal renal, adrenal, thyroid, cardiac and liver
e) Euvolaemic on examination

SIADH can occur in a vast range of conditions including pneumonia, malignancy, mesothelioma, subarachnoid haemorrhage amongst other diseases.

Although conventional management of SIADH requires fluid restriction, often to 800ml to 1L/day, it is always imperative to stop the offending drugs first; in this case, furosemide and ramipril, as these can persistently lower serum sodium.

Increasing the levothyroxine is unlikely to create a major impact given that the patient's TSH is within the normal range. If the TSH was elevated, then this may be an option. Failure of fluid restriction may merit a trial of demeclocycline, which impairs the action of ADH, although this may soon be superseded by a novel class of ADH receptor antagonists (vaptans).

Hoorn EJ, van der Lubbe N and Zietse R. SIADH and hyponatraemia: why does it matter? NDT Plus. 2009. 2[Suppl 3]: iii5-iii 11.

22) B: Gliclazide

Under normal circumstances, the drug of choice for type 2 diabetes in overweight patients is metformin. However, when creatinine is more than 150 micromol/l (or eGFR< 30ml/min/1,73m^2), metformin is absolutely contraindicated as it increases the risk of lactic acidosis. Pioglitazone is contraindicated due to the history of heart failure. Sulphonylureas are the most appropriate treatment, preferably shorter acting forms (i.e. gliclazide). Long acting sulphonylureas, such as glibenclamide should be avoided as they carry a greater risk of hypoglycaemia.

National Institute for Health and Clinical Excellence. 2008. Type 2 diabetes. CG 66 London: National Institute for Health and Clinical Excellence.

23) A: Inhibits hepatic gluconeogenesis

Option A) correctly describes the action of metformin. Sulphonylureas work by stimulating insulin secretion. They achieve this by inhibiting ATP-activated potassium channels on the beta cells of the islet of Langerhans. This results in depolarisation and activation of calcium channels. The calcium ion influx stimulates exocytosis of granules containing insulin. Pioglitazone works by stimulating peroxisome proliferator-activated receptor gamma (PPAR-gamma), but they also activate PPAR-alpha receptors to a lesser extent. The DPP-IV inhibitors include the gliptins, and they work by reducing the breakdown of incretins (e.g. GLP-1).

24) B: Magnesium

Serum magnesium must always be measured in patients with resistant hypokalaemia as failure to correct magnesium deficiency will result in failure to correct potassium deficiency. Patients with chronic alcohol excess are frequently malnourished and are often deficient in multiple vitamins and minerals.

25) D: 360

The plasma osmolality can be calculated by the following equation:

$$\text{Plasma osmolality (mOsm/kg)} = 2Na + Urea + Glucose$$
$$= 2(150) + 15 + 45$$
$$= 360 \text{ mOsm/kg}$$

26) E) Intravenous fluid resuscitation

Diabetic ketoacidosis (DKA) is a medical emergency requiring prompt recognition and treatment. It is often triggered by intercurrent illness. This patient has sepsis secondary to a community-acquired pneumonia. Patients with DKA are very dehydrated with a total fluid deficit of around 100ml/kg, thus making IV fluid resuscitation the most important treatment measure.

Diagnosis of DKA is made by identifying the presence of all three of the following:

a)   Capillary glucose > 11mol/l
b)   Capillary ketones >3mmol/l or urinary ketones 2+ or more
c)   Venous pH < 7.3 and/or bicarbonate <15 mmol/l

Treatment requires gaining IV access, taking bloods (including FBC, U and E, plasma glucose and venous blood gas), commencing IV fluids (successive 1L bags given over 30 minutes, 1hourly, 2hourly, 2hourly, then 4 to 6 hourly) and starting a fixed rate insulin infusion of 0.1 units/kg/hr. In cases of sepsis triggering DKA, blood cultures should be taken and appropriate intravenous antibiotics administered. 12-lead ECGs should routinely be performed in any acutely ill patient.

BMs, ketones, venous bicarbonate and electrolytes should be monitored at frequent intervals. Regularly measuring potassium is imperative as the insulin will continue to drive potassium ions into the cells. If the potassium is not replaced accordingly, patients can quickly become hypokalaemic. Once the metabolic acidosis, ketonaemia and hyperglycaemia are corrected, and once the patient starts eating and drinking, the fixed rate insulin infusion can be stopped. Importantly, the patient should be given their regular subcutaneous insulin dose 30 minutes to 1 hour before the insulin infusion has been stopped. This will provide enough time for the effects of the short-acting subcutaneous insulin to kick in, whilst the IV insulin wears off, and thus prevent a potential reoccurrence of DKA.

In reality, therefore, options b) to e) all form an integral part of the immediate management of DKA and should be performed within quick succession of each other. If biochemical resolution is achieved (i.e. Ketones < 0.3, pH > 7.3) and the patient is not ready to eat or drink, the patient can be switched to a variable rate sliding scale insulin infusion.

Savage MW, Dhatariya KK, Kilvert A et al. Diabetes UK Position Statements and Care Recommendations. Joint British Diabetes Societies Guidelines for the Management of Diabetic Ketoacidosis. Diabetic Medicine. 2011; 28: 508-15.

27) C: Plasma osmolality should be corrected at a rate of 10-14 mOsm/kg/hour

The patient has presented with Hyperosmolar Hyperglycaemic State (HHS). The diagnosis is made when patients, often with a background of type 2 diabetes, present with the following:

1) Generally unwell and severe dehydration
2) Plasma osmolality > 320 mOsm/kg
3) Plasma glucose > 30 mmol/l **without** significant hyperketonaemia (<3 mmol/l), ketonuria (2+ or less) or acidosis (pH>7.3, bicarbonate >15 mmol/l)

HHS is clinically and biochemically distinct from diabetic ketoacidosis (DKA) and accordingly requires a different management approach.

HHS tends to affect patients with type 2 diabetes whilst DKA affects those with type1 diabetes (although advanced type 2 diabetics who are absolutely insulin deficient are also susceptible to DKA). HHS has a higher mortality then DKA, partly because it predominantly affects older patients with multiple co-morbidities. HHS patients are more severely dehydrated than those with DKA, often presenting with a fluid deficit of 100-220ml/kg and typically a more marked hyperglycaemia. Despite these distinctions, patients can indeed develop a mixed DKA/HHS-type picture.

As with DKA, IV fluid resuscitation is the most important aspect of managing HHS; not only will this correct dehydration, but it will help lower serum glucose levels. Plasma osmolality should be corrected at a rate of around 3-8 mOsm/kg/hour – excessive corrections can result in rapid shifts of fluid in different body compartments, which can potentially lead to severe complications including cerebral oedema and central pontine myelinolysis. If there is evidence of hyperketonaemia (3-beta-hydroxybutyrate serum levels >1 mmol/l), a fixed rate insulin infusion of 0.05units/kg/hour (half the rate in DKA) should be started immediately. However, if there is no hyperketonaemia, this insulin infusion should only be given once IV fluid resuscitation no longer lowers plasma glucose at the desired rate (aim for a rate of fall in plasma glucose of 3-5 mmol/l/hour). Once BMs are less than 10-15 and the patient starts to eat and drink, stop the insulin infusion and recommence the patient's usual anti-diabetic medication.

Joint British Diabetes Societies Inpatient Care Group. The management of the hyperosmolar hyperglycaemic state (HHS) in adults with diabetes. August 2012.

O'Malley G, Moran C, Draman MS et al. Central pontine myelinolysis complicating treatment of the hyperglycaemic hyperosmolar state. Annals of Clinical Biochemistry. 2008; 45:440-3.

28) A: Short synacthen test

The short synacthen test involves measuring serum cortisol, then administering 250 micrograms of synthetic ACTH (tetracosactide) intravenously/intramuscularly followed by another measurement of serum cortisol 30 and 60 minutes later. If the cortisol fails to rise to more than 500nmol/l at 30 or 60 minutes, then the patient is likely to have Addison's disease. Measuring random serum cortisol is of little use due to its diurnal variation (reaching a peak in the early morning and a trough at midnight).

29) D: 6-8 litres

Patients with DKA are often very dehydrated and require prompt fluid resuscitation. The fluid deficit in DKA is around 100ml/kg, so in a 70kg male, the answer is approximately 7 litres.

Trachtenbarg DE. Diabetic Ketoacidosis. American Family Physician. 2005;71:1705-14

30) E: 21-alpha hydroxylase

The diagnosis is congenital adrenal hyperplasia (CAH), of which multiple clinical variants exist. The most common enzyme deficiency causing CAH is 21-alpha hydroxylase, which is ultimately required for the synthesis of cortisol and aldosterone. Deficient enzyme activity not only causes cortisol and aldosterone depletion, but the precursor molecules become diverted towards the synthesis of androgens (e.g. testosterone and dihydrotesterone).

In classical CAH, there is severe 21-alpha hydroxylase deficiency causing presentation in early childhood with salt-wasting crises, dehydration, vomiting and failure to thrive. Female neonates have ambiguous genitalia secondary to in utero exposure to high circulating androgens.

Milder forms of CAH can present later in childhood with precocious puberty. Even milder variants can present in adulthood with hirsutism, oligomenorrhoea and infertility.

Speiser PW and White PC. Congenital Adrenal Hyperplasia. The New England Journal of Medicine. 2003;349: 776-88

31) D: Zona fasciculata

The inner adrenal medulla secretes catecholamines. The outer adrenal cortex is histologically divided into 3 zones. These are, from peripheral to central:

a) Zona glomerulosa – produces mineralocorticoids
b) Zona fasciculata – produces glucocorticoids
c) Zona reticularis – produces sex steroids

32) A: Pseudo-Cushing's syndrome

Cushing's syndrome is the clinical state associated with chronic glucocorticoid excess. It is most commonly iatrogenic, secondary to chronic exposure to exogenous steroids, but is less frequently associated with excessive endogenous steroid production. Approximately 80%

of endogenous causes of Cushing's syndrome is secondary to an ACTH-secreting pituitary adenoma (i.e. Cushing's disease), and the remaining 20% are due to ectopic ACTH-producing tumours (e.g. from small cell lung carcinomas).

Clinical features of Cushing's syndrome include central obesity, acne, buffalo hump, supraclavicular fat pad, hypertension and cognitive disorders (e.g. depression, psychosis, short term memory problems) amongst others. However, all these symptoms and signs are relatively non-specific and can form part of the pseudo-Cushing's syndrome (i.e. the Cushingoid phenotype associated with conditions such as obesity, chronic alcohol excess and type 2 diabetes). More discriminative features of Cushing's syndrome span wide abdominal striae, facial plethora, proximal myopathy and easy bruising.

When a diagnosis of Cushing's syndrome is suspected, certain investigations should be pursued, which include:

a) *24-hour urinary free cortisol or late night salivary cortisol* – these are useful screening tests for Cushing's syndrome. However, false-positive results can occur in pseudo-Cushing's syndrome.

b) *Low dose dexamethasone suppression test* – this involves giving 0.5mg of dexamethasone every 6 hours for 48 hours and measuring urine and serum cortisol at 0 and 48 hours. A positive test result is when dexamethasone fails to suppress free cortisol levels, and helps confirm a diagnosis of Cushing's syndrome, whilst excluding pseudo-Cushing's.

c) *High dose dexamethasone suppression test* – this involves giving 2mg dexamethasone every 6 hours for 48 hours and measuring urine and serum cortisol at 0 and 48 hours. Failure to suppress serum cortisol with these high doses of dexamethasone suggests an ectopic rather pituitary source of ACTH, as the pituitary still retains some negative feedback control, unlike ectopic sources.

Nieman LK, Biller BMK, Findling JW et al. The Diagnosis of Cushing's Syndrome: An Endocrine Society Clinical Practise Guideline. The Journal of Clinical Endocrinology & Metabolism. 2008; 93: 1526-40

33) E: Bilateral inferior petrosal sinus sampling

After confirming the presence of Cushing's syndrome, it is important to identify the location of the source driving this pathology. Measuring serum ACTH levels is very useful in this regard. If serum ACTH levels are undetectable, a cortisol-secreting adrenal source is likely (usually an adrenal adenoma), as this will suppress ACTH production from the anterior pituitary, indicating the need for imaging the adrenals. However, if serum ACTH is detectable, then the Cushing's syndrome is either secondary to a pituitary or ectopic source. As discussed previously, a high dose dexamethasone suppression test will help to differentiate the two, but this is not the gold standard test.

An MRI of the pituitary gland will fail to detect ACTH-secreting pituitary micro-adenomas due to the limited resolution of this imaging. However, sampling the inferior petrosal sinuses (where the pituitary gland drains) for ACTH, and finding high levels of inferior petrosal sinus ACTH compared with the systemic circulation, confirms the pituitary source – this is the gold standard investigation.

Findling JW and Raff H. Clinical Review: Cushing's Syndrome: Important Issues in Diagnosis and Management. The Journal of Clinical Endocrinology & Metabolism. 2006; 91: 3746-53

34) E: Measure plasma glucose at 3-5am over several nights and adjust insulin glargine accordingly

The patient's main problem resides in controlling his fasting morning plasma glucose hence starting a basal bolus regimen is not required. Although at first sight it may seem reasonable to increase his long-acting insulin at night (glargine), a fasting morning hyperglycaemia may not necessarily be secondary to under-dosing of the previous night's insulin. In fact, if the long-acting insulin taken at night is over-dosed, the patient may develop a period of hypoglycaemia during the early hours of the morning, activating stress hormones and subsequently inducing a rebound morning hyperglycaemia.

This phenomenon is called the Somogyi effect, and the most appropriate solution is to exclude the possibility of this early morning hypoglycaemia by measuring BMs at 3-5am and adjusting the long-acting insulin accordingly. If the patient becomes hypoglycaemic during this period, the glargine should be reduced.

35) A: Stein-Leventhal syndrome

The most likely diagnosis is polycystic ovarian syndrome (PCOS), otherwise known as Stein-Leventhal syndrome. The diagnosis is made when at least 2 out of the 3 of the following are present:

a) Clinical or biochemical evidence of hyperandrogenism
b) Oligomenorrhoea or amenorrhoea
c) Polycystic ovaries on ultrasound

Patients with PCOS are typically overweight, often having a metabolic syndrome-type phenotype (type II diabetes, hypertension, hypercholesterolaemia, obesity). 24-hour urinary free cortisol is thus likely to be elevated as discussed previously, representing a pseudo-Cushing's syndrome. LH is often elevated, whilst FSH can be normal or low; an LH to FSH of approximately 2:1 or 3:1 is highly suggestive of PCOS.

Option E) is incorrect as an androgen-secreting tumour would produce significantly greater levels of serum testosterone. Although late-onset congenital adrenal hyperplasia can present with similar symptoms and signs as PCOS, it is far less common.

Weight loss is the most effective treatment for PCOS. If this fails, then patients may be given a trial of metformin. This will not only reduce insulin resistance, which is often ubiquitous to this syndrome, but will also help improve fertility.

Ehrmann DA. Polycystic Ovary Syndrome. The New England Journal of Medicine. 2005;352: 1223-36

36) A: Androgen insensitivity syndrome

Patients with androgen insensitivity syndrome (AIS) (also known as testicular feminisation) have the appearance of female external genitalia, but are genetically male. The pathophysiology is driven by a mutation in the androgen receptor gene, resulting in a failure of cell response to circulating androgens in utero. AIS patients have testes, but these fail to develop and descend down the inguinal canal, explaining the history of bilateral indirect inguinal hernia repairs during childhood.

Patients with Klinefelter's syndrome have the XXY karyotype, are phenotypically male and typically have a tall stature. Turner's syndrome patients have a single X chromosome. Kallmann syndrome is the combination of hypogonadotrophic hypogonadism and congenital anosmia. Noonan's syndrome patients are phenotypically male, but share many other clinical features with Turner's syndrome.

Practise Committee of American Society for Reproductive Medicine. Current evaluation of amenorrhea. Fertility and Sterility. 2008;90: S219-25.

37) C: Hypocalcaemia

Nephrogenic diabetes (renal resistance to ADH) can be caused by lithium therapy, hypokalaemia and hypercalcaemia (not hypocalcaemia). Hyperglycaemia produces an osmotic diuresis, whilst cranial diabetes insipidus involves a lack of ADH production. Making a diagnosis of diabetes insipidus requires undertaking the water deprivation test. Patients with this condition tend to produce copious amounts of urine (>3L/day) and can rapidly become dehydrated.

Makaryus AN and McFarlane SI. Diabetes insipidus: Diagnosis and treatment of a complex disease. Cleveland Clinic Journal of Medicine. 2006;73: 65-71.

38) C: 7.5mg

Prednisolone is 4 times more potent than hydrocortisone and has a longer duration of action. Thus, 30mg of hydrocortisone is equivalent to 7.5mg of prednisolone. Note that the doses of steroid therapy given in glucocorticoid deficiency is designed to grossly mimic the natural diurnal rhythm, by giving two-thirds of the dose in the morning and one-third in the evening.

British Medical Association and the Royal Pharmaceutical Society of Great Britain. British National Formulary. 62nd ed. UK: BMJ Publishing Group. 2011.

39) A: Hypocalcaemia

A common risk of thyroid surgery includes accidental destruction of the parathyroid glands. This leads to primary hypoparathyroidism and consequent hypocalcaemia. Typical symptoms include perioral tingling and numbness, muscle spasms and in severe cases, seizures and laryngospasm. Signs to elicit in hypocalcaemia include Chvostek's and Trousseau's sign. Chvostek's sign is positive when tapping the cheek over the parotid in the region of the facial nerve induces ipsilateral muscle twitching. Trousseau's sign is positive when inflating a blood pressure cuff around a patients arm induces carpopedal spasm.

Cooper MS and Gittoes NJL. Diagnosis and management of hypocalcaemia. British Medical Journal. 2008;336: 1298-1302

40) B: Raloxifene works as an oestrogen receptor agonist

Osteoporosis is characterised by reduced bone mass and compromised micro-architectural quality. The WHO definition of osteoporosis is a bone mineral density (BMD) of 2.5 standard deviations or more below normal peak bone mass of a young adult (i.e. T score ≤ -2.5). A T-score of between -1 and -2.5 is osteopenia.

Vertebral crush fractures, Colles fractures and fractured neck of femurs following minimal impact should all raise suspicion of osteoporosis.

Raloxifene is used in the prevention of osteoporosis in postmenopausal women. It works as a selective oestrogen receptor modulator, behaving as an oestrogen receptor agonist in bone and uterus, but an oestrogen receptor antagonist in breast. Secondary causes of osteoporosis include thyrotoxicosis, hypogonadism and Cushing's syndrome.

Poole KES and Compston JE. Osteoporosis and its management. British Medical Journal. 2006;333: 1251-6.

Respiratory Questions

1) A 64-year old man who has recently returned from a business holiday, having stayed in a hotel, presents with a 5-day history of headache, dyspnoea, dry cough and diarrhoea.

   On examination he is febrile (temp. 38.4 degrees Celsius), heart rate 78/min regular, BP 142/78mmHg and respiratory rate of 22/min. Investigations are as follows:

Haemoglobin	12.4g/dl (11.5-13.5)
WCC	14.8 x10^9/l (3.5-9)
Platelets	420 x 10^9/l (140-400)
Na$^+$	130mmol/l (135-145)
K$^+$	4.2 mmol/l (3.5-5.5)
Urea	7.2 mmol/l (2.5-7.5)
Creatinine	98 micromol/l (40-90)
Aspartate Transaminase (AST)	220 U/L (5-45)
Alkaline Phosphatase (ALP)	180 U/L (25-110)

   Chest X-Ray – Bilateral patchy consolidation with a right-sided pleural effusion

   Which of the following antibiotics represents first-line management?

   A. Ciprofloxacin
   B. Doxycycline
   C. Co-amoxiclav
   D. Benzylpenicillin
   E. Clarithromycin

2) A 25-year old man presents with a 2-week history of dyspnoea, left-sided pleuritic chest pain, dry cough, myalgia and painful shins. He is otherwise fit and well with no significant past medical history.

   On examination, his temperature is 38.3 degrees Celsius, pulse 76/min and regular and BP of 118/76 mmHg.

Investigations reveal a normocytic anaemia with an Hb of 9.6g/dl (11.4-14). Blood film reveals evidence of schistocytosis and a Chest X-ray shows consolidation in the left lower lobe. Cold agglutinin test is positive.

Which of the following represents the most likely causative micro-organism?

A. Staphylococcus aureus
B. Legionella pneumophila
C. Mycoplasma pneumoniae
D. Streptococcus pneumoniae
E. Chlamydophila pneumoniae

3) A 30-year old otherwise fit and healthy male presents to the emergency department with sudden onset breathlessness and right-sided pleuritic chest pain. The patient is haemodynamically stable.

A chest X-ray confirms a right-sided pneumothorax with a rim of 3cm.

What is the most appropriate initial management?

A. Insert a chest drain in the 2nd intercostal space, mid-clavicular line
B. Aspirate with a 16-18 G cannula
C. Aspirate with a 20-22G cannula
D. Observe
E. Insert a chest drain in the 5th intercostal space, mid-axillary line

4) A 34-year old female presents to the emergency department with a 3-day history of progressive dyspnoea and cough productive of green sputum. On examination, her respiratory rate is 28/min, heart rate 120/min, BP 106/74mmHg, temperature 38.4 degrees Celsius and GCS 15/15. Bloods are as follows:

Haemoglobin (Hb)	13.6g/dl (11.4-14)	Na$^+$	144 mmol/l (135-145)
White Cells	13.4 x10^9/l (3.5-9)	K$^+$	3.8 mmol/l (3.5-5.0)

Neutrophils	$10 \times 10^9/l$ (1.2-7.7)	Urea	6.8 mmol/l (2.5-7.5)
Platelets	$540 \times 10^9/l$ (150-400)	Creatinine	76 micromol/l (40-90)

C-reactive Peptide (CRP) 180 (1-10)

Which of the following is the patient's CURB-65 score?

A. 0
B. 1
C. 2
D. 3
E. 4

5) A 54-year old homeless male presents to the medical assessment unit with a 4-day history of fevers, rigors and a cough productive of purulent sputum.

He has a history of chronic alcohol abuse consuming approximately 36 units per week.

On examination, he was febrile with a temperature of 38.8 degrees Celsius. There was dullness to percussion, increased tactile vocal fremitus and bronchial breathing in the region of the left apex.

A Chest X-ray shows consolidation in the left upper zone with some cavitation.

Which of the following is the most likely diagnosis?

A. Klebsiella pneumonia
B. Aspiration pneumonia
C. Mycoplasma pneumonia
D. Legionella pneumonia
E. Primary Tuberculosis

6) Which of the following is NOT a respiratory cause of digital clubbing?

   A. Cryptogenic fibrosing alveolitis
   B. Cystic fibrosis
   C. Bronchiectasis
   D. Malignant mesothelioma
   E. Chronic obstructive pulmonary disease

7) A patient known to have COPD is reviewed in the chest clinic. His physician calculates his FEV1 % predicted, and finds that his patient has severe COPD.

Which of the following FEV1% predicted does this correspond too?

   A. ≥ 80%
   B. 50-79%
   C. 40-59%
   D. 30-49%
   E. < 30%

8) A patient with poorly controlled COPD sees his GP complaining of on-going shortness of breath and cough with minimal relief from PRN salbutamol.

After undergoing spirometry, it is discovered that his FEV1 is 65% of that predicted for his age, sex and height.

Which of the following medications should be added to his current regimen?

   A. Ipratropium inhaler
   B. Seretide 250 accuhaler
   C. Seretide 500 accuhaler
   D. Tiotropium inhaler
   E. Tiotropium and salmeterol

9) A 20-year old female student presents to the emergency department with acute onset shortness of breath. She is diagnosed as having an acute exacerbation of her asthma.

She is unable to complete sentences in one breath and has a respiratory rate of 30 breaths per minute. Her pulse is 120 beats/minute and systolic oxygen saturations are 94% on air.

Her peak expiratory flow rate is recorded at 33% of predicted.

Which of her clinical features is not a recognised feature of acute severe asthma?

A. PEF 33% predicted
B. Unable to complete short sentences in one breath
C. Respiratory rate > 25/min
D. Pulse rate > 110 beats/minute
E. Oxygen saturations 94%

10) A 19-year old female is treated in the Emergency Department for an acute severe asthma attack. She has been given high flow oxygen, nebulised bronchodilators and IV hydrocortisone.

Despite these treatments, she remains significantly short of breath.

Which of the following represents the next most appropriate line of management?

A. IV Magnesium 1.2-2g over 20 minutes
B. Arterial blood gas and titrate oxygen accordingly
C. IV aminophylline
D. IV Magnesium 0.5 – 1g over 20 minutes
E. IV salbutamol

11) A 92-year old gentleman with known COPD presents to the medical assessment unit with a 3-day history of increasing shortness of breath and cough productive of purulent sputum.

His past medical history includes ischaemic heart disease, congestive cardiac failure and chronic kidney disease. Despite receiving controlled oxygen therapy, maintaining his SaO2 at 88-92%, nebulised salbutamol and ipratropium, prednisolone and IV augmentin, he continues to remain significantly short of breath.

An arterial blood gas is repeated with an FiO2 of 28%, which is as follows:

pH	7.32 (7.35-7.45)
PaO_2	7.0kPa (11-13)
$PaCO_2$	7.2kPa (4.7-7.0)
HCO_3^-	32 mEq/L (22-26)

Which of the following is the next most appropriate treatment?

A. Intubation and ventilation
B. Lower FiO2 to 24%
C. Trial of non-invasive ventilation
D. Observe and repeat ABG in 20-30 mins
E. IV hydrocortisone stat

12) A 35-year old woman presents with a 1-month history of progressive dyspnoea, dry cough and malaise. She is of African-American origin but has no past medical history of note.

Examination findings include an indurated, violaceous plaque on the left side of the nose and cheek and an irregularly shaped left pupil.

Observations are temperature 37.2 degrees Celsius, BP 124/74mmHg, heart rate 84 regular and respiratory rate 24/min.

A chest X-ray shows bilateral hilar lymphadenopathy.

Which of the following is INCORRECT regarding this condition?

A. Bilateral hilar lymphadenopathy only, on the chest X-ray represents stage 1 of the disease
B. Lupus pernio is a poor prognostic indicator of the condition
C. The histological hallmark of the disease is non-caseating granulomatous formation
D. Serum ACE is raised in approximately 20% of patients
E. Cranial-nerve palsies represents the most common neurological manifestation

13) Which of the following conditions is NOT preferentially associated with upper lobe pulmonary fibrosis?

A. Extrinsic allergic alveolitis
B. Tuberculosis
C. Ankylosing spondylitis
D. Sarcoidosis
E. Asbestosis

14) For which of the following patients with sarcoidosis is oral steroid therapy NOT absolutely indicated?

A. 33-year old female with anterior uveitis refractory to topical steroid treatment
B. 22-year old male with right sided facial palsy
C. 32-year old male with an adjusted calcium of 2.8
D. 35-year old female with cardiac sarcoidosis and evidence of ECG abnormalities
E. 28-year old male found to have bilateral hilar lymphadenopathy and pulmonary infiltrates on the chest X –ray

15) A 23-year old student with asthma sees his GP due to persistent shortness of breath limiting his exercise tolerance.

He is currently taking PRN salbutamol inhalers, 400 micrograms of beclomethasone inhaler per day and reports that he was recently started on a salmeterol inhaler for which he has derived no benefit.

His GP decides to step up his asthma treatment.

According to British Thoracic Society (BTS) guidelines, which of the following represents the most appropriate next-line management?

A. Continue salmeterol and increase beclomethasone to 800 micrograms/day
B. Continue salmeterol and increase beclomethasone to 2000 micrograms/day
C. Stop salmeterol and increase beclomethasone to 800 micrograms/day
D. Stop salmeterol and add in a leukotriene receptor antagonist
E. Stop salmeterol and add in SR theophylline

16) Which of the following chest malignancies is most commonly associated with hypercalcaemia?

A. Small cell lung carcinoma
B. Large cell lung carcinoma
C. Squamous cell lung carcinoma
D. Adenocarcinoma of the lung
E. Malignant mesothelioma

17) A 73-year old gentleman is reviewed by the chest physician in clinic. The patient complains of a 2-month history of progressive loss of appetite, weight loss, lethargy, dyspnoea and cough.

He is an ex-smoker with a 40-pack year history.

Examination findings are unremarkable. Investigations are as follows:

Haemoglobin	12.8g/dl (11.5-14.0)	Na⁺	126 mmol/l (135-145)
Mean Cell Volume (MCV)	84fl (84-95)	K⁺	4.0 mmol/l (3.5-5)
Platelets	440 x10⁹/l (140-400)	Urea	4.2 mmol/l (60-120)
White Cell Count	10 x10⁹/l (3.5-9)	Creat	80 mmol/l (40-90)

Paired serum and urine osmolalities = 264 mOsm/kg and 240 mOsm/kg respectively
(serum 280-295; urine 300-900)

Urine Sodium 40 mmol/l
Random serum cortisol is 480
Thyroid and liver function tests are normal.

Chest X-ray = 3cm opacification in the left midzone

Which of the following histological subtypes of cancers is the most likely diagnosis?

A. Squamous cell lung carcinoma
B. Large cell lung carcinoma
C. Adenocarcinoma of the lung
D. Small cell lung carcinoma
E. Malignant mesothelioma

18) You are asked to perform a respiratory examination on a patient. You find that there is dullness to percussion, reduced breath sounds, reduced vocal resonance and reduced tactile vocal fremitus on the right base of the chest.

A pleural tap is performed by your registrar, who sends a sample for biochemical analysis, the results of which are as follows:

Pleural fluid protein   37g/L
Pleural fluid: serum protein   0.8
LDH pleural: serum ratio   0.7
Which of the following diagnoses is least likely?

A. Empyema
B. Lung malignancy
C. Tuberculosis
D. Rheumatoid arthritis
E. Nephrotic syndrome

19) A 78-year old male presents to his GP complaining of a 5-month history of progressively worsening breathlessness and reduced exercise tolerance. He is a retired shipyard worker.

On examination, there is evidence of finger clubbing and fine bilateral inspiratory crackles.

What is the most likely diagnosis?

A. Idiopathic Pulmonary Fibrosis
B. Asbestosis
C. Silicosis
D. Berylliosis
E. Siderosis

20) What is the average latency period between asbestos exposure and the development of malignant mesothelioma?

A. 3-6 months
B. 6-12 months
C. 3-5 years
D. 5-10 years
E. 20-35 years

21) Which of the following is the correct definition for the term PaO_2?

A. Partial pressure of oxygen combined with arterial haemoglobin
B. Partial pressure of oxygen dissolved in arterial plasma
C. Partial pressure of oxygen in the alveoli
D. Partial pressure of oxygen in the airways
E. Partial pressure of oxygen in venous plasma

22) Which of the following case scenarios is NOT considered a major risk factor for thromboembolic disease?

A. 26-year old lady who is 34 weeks pregnant
B. 25-year old patient known ulcerative colitis who is 3 days post-colectomy for toxic megacolon
C. 73-year old lady who is 4 days post-right hemi-arthroplasty for a fractured neck of femur
D. 54-year old male with renal cell carcinoma and pulmonary metastases
E. 24-year old lady on the combined oral contraceptive pill

23) You are the junior doctor on-call and you get bleeped by a nurse who asks you to review a medical patient complaining of sudden onset shortness of breath.

She is a 58-year old lady admitted 3 days previously with dyspnoea and cough, for which a diagnosis of lobar pneumonia was made.

The patient is known to have squamous cell carcinoma of the lung with bony metastases. Since admission, she has received 2 full days of intravenous antibiotics, which were switched to oral yesterday. An entry made during the most recent ward round suggests that the patient's breathlessness and mobility has progressively improved during her stay in hospital.

On questioning the patient, she complains of sudden onset worsening of breathlessness and denies any chest pain.

On examination, the patient is dyspnoeic at rest, respiratory rate is 26/min, heart rate is 120/min and regular, BP is stable at 124/82 mmHg, SaO2 has recently dropped from 96% to 92% on air.

You perform an ABG on air, which reveals the following:

pH	7.47 (7.35-7.45)
PaO_2	7.6 kPa (11-13)
$PaCO_2$	4.2 kPa (4.7-6.0)
HCO_3^-	22 mEq/L (22-26)

After administering high flow oxygen, which of the following is the most appropriate management plan? (Assuming that the patient weighs 80kg)

A. Arrange a CT Pulmonary Angiogram (CTPA) and, if positive, commence warfarin with 120mg daily enoxaparin. Stop enoxaparin once INR > 2

B. Give 80mg enoxaparin, arrange a CTPA and, if positive, start warfarin with the enoxaparin to be stopped once INR >2

C. Give 120mg enoxaparin, arrange a CTPA and, if positive, start warfarin with the enoxaparin to be stopped once the INR>2

D. Give 120mg enoxaparin, arrange a CTPA and, if positive, continue daily 120mg enoxaparin lifelong

E. Give 80mg enoxaparin, arrange a CTPA and, if positive, continue daily 80mg enoxaparin lifelong

24) A 64-year old man presents to Accident and Emergency with pleuritic chest pain and shortness of breath. He recently returned from a holiday in Australia.

What is the gold-standard investigation for his condition?

A. Pulmonary arteriography
B. CT pulmonary angiography (CTPA)
C. Ventilation-perfusion scan (V/Q scan)
D. D-dimer
E. Venous doppler USS

25) A 42-year old lady presents with a 2-week history of progressive shortness of breath, dry cough and decreased exercise tolerance. Her past medical history includes type 1 diabetes, hypertension and right renal transplant 1 year previously. The patient is allergic to trimethoprim, with a history of anaphylaxis.

On examination, chest is clear and heart sounds are normal. Observations are heart rate 106/min regular, respiratory rate 22/min, temperature 37.9 degrees Celsius and oxygen saturation 94% on air at rest.

You note that as the patient transfers from bed to chair, saturations drop to 82% on air.

Investigations are as follows:

Haemoglobin (Hb)	13.4g/dl (11.5-14.0)	Na$^+$ 136 mmol/l (135-145)
White Cell Count	9.4 x 10^9/l (4-9)	K$^+$ 4.2 mmol/l (3.5-5.0)
Neutrophils	3.2 x10^9/l (1.2-7.7)	Urea 4.6 mmol/l (2.5-7.5)
Platelets	402 x10^9/l (150-400)	Creat 100 micromol/l (40-90)

Chest X ray = Bilateral perihilar interstitial shadowing

Which of the following is the most appropriate treatment?

A. High dose septrin (co-trimoxazole)
B. IV pentamidine
C. Clarithromycin
D. IV hydrocortisone
E. Amphotericin B

26) Which of the following drugs is NOT a recognised cause of pulmonary fibrosis?

A. Methotrexate
B. Amiodarone
C. Busulphan
D. Nitrofurantoin
E. Amlodipine

27) An elderly lady with rheumatoid arthritis is reviewed in the rheumatology clinic. She complains of a 6-week history of dry cough and worsening shortness of breath.

The attending physician suspects a case of pulmonary fibrosis.

Which of the following examination findings on auscultation of the chest is most consistent with this diagnosis?

A. Bilateral basal fine early inspiratory crackles
B. Bilateral basal fine late inspiratory crackles
C. Bilateral basal coarse early inspiratory crackles
D. Bilateral basal coarse late inspiratory crackles
E. Unilateral fine early inspiratory crackles

28) A 67-year old male presents to the emergency department with a 5-day history of shortness of breath, productive cough and right-sided pleuritic chest pain. He is disorientated in place and time.

On examination there is reduced air entry and bronchial breathing in the right base.

Respiratory rate is 32/min, blood pressure is 100/76 mmHg, heart rate is 98/min and temperature is 38.3 degrees.

Investigations are as follows:

Haemoglobin	12.2g/dl (11.5-14.0)
White Cell Count	17.8 x10^9/l (3-9)
Neutrophils	12.2 x10^9/l (1.2-7)
Platelets	584 x10^9/l (15-400)
Na$^+$	136 mmol/l (135-145)
K$^+$	3.8 mmol/l (3.5-5.0)
Urea	10.2 mmol/l (2-7)
Creat	68 micromol/l (40-90)
C-reactive Peptide	304 (<10)

Chest X-ray = right lower lobe consolidation

Which of the following is the most appropriate first-line antibiotic treatment?

A. Oral co-amoxiclav 625mg TDS
B. Oral amoxicillin 500mg TDS and oral clarithromycin 500mg BD
C. Intravenous ciprofloxacin 500mg BD
D. Intravenous co-amoxiclav 1.2g TDS and oral clarithromycin 500mg BD
E. Intravenous co-amoxiclav 1.2g TDS

29) Which of the following arterial blood gas results is most consistent with chronic type II respiratory failure in a patient with severe chronic obstructive pulmonary disease?

A. pH 7.02, PaO_2 13.40, $PaCO_2$ 3.80, HCO_3 7.11
B. pH 7.38, PaO_2 7.60, $PaCO_2$ 5.1, HCO_3 22.00
C. pH 7.50, PaO_2 14.02, $PaCO_2$ 3.9, HCO_3 22.04
D. pH 7.35, PaO_2 6.8, $PaCO_2$ 8.4, HCO_3 33.61
E. pH 7.34, PaO_2 6.6, $PaCO_2$ 8.6, HCO_3 24.02

30) Which of the following patients would NOT qualify for long-term oxygen therapy (LTOT) according to British Thoracic Society guidelines?

A. 73-year old male with bronchiectasis and a PaO_2, which is consistently 7.4kPa on air
B. 84-year old female with chronic heart failure and a PaO_2, which is consistently 6.8kPa on air
C. 81-year old male with chronic obstructive pulmonary disease who has a PaO_2, which is consistently 7.6kPa on air, and pulmonary hypertension
D. 38-year old female with cystic fibrosis who has a PaO_2, which is consistently 7.8kPa on air, and secondary polycythaemia
E. 75-year old male with cryptogenic fibrosing alveolitis who has a PaO_2, which is consistently 7.1kPa on air

31) A 42-year old male who has recently emigrated from Nigeria presents to his GP with a 4-week history of cough, night sweats, weight loss and loss of appetite. A chest X-ray shows cavitating lesions in the upper lobes bilaterally.

Which of the following is the most likely diagnosis?

A. Primary Tuberculosis
B. Progressive Primary Tuberculosis
C. Secondary Tuberculosis
D. Miliary Tuberculosis
E. Lymphoma

32) Which of the following represents the first-line chemotherapy regimen for pulmonary tuberculosis?

A. Isoniazid and rifampicin for first 4 months, then pyrazinamide and ethambutol for subsequent 2 months
B. Rifampicin, isoniazid, pyrazinamide and ethambutol for 6 months
C. Isoniazid and rifampicin for 6 months, supplemented by pyrazinamide and ethambutol for the first 2 months
D. Isoniazid and rifampicin for 6 months, supplemented by pyrazinamide and ethambutol for the first 4 months
E. Rifampicin and pyrazinamide for 6 months, supplemented by isoniazid and ethambutol for the first 2 months

33) Which of the following anti-tuberculosis drugs is most likely to affect the optic nerve?

A. Rifampicin
B. Isoniazid
C. Pyrazinamide
D. Ethambutol
E. Streptomycin

34) Which of the following is INCORRECT regarding cystic fibrosis (CF)?

A. It is caused by a mutation in the CFTR gene in chromosome 13
B. Approximately 15% of infants with CF are born with meconium ileus
C. 85-90% of infants develop pancreatic insufficiency
D. Virtually all men with classic CF are infertile because of congenital bilateral absence of the vas deferens
E. Cystic fibrosis affects roughly 1 in 3000 births in those of Northern European decent.

35) A 56-year old gentleman who is day 7 post-open right hemicolectomy is reviewed on the ward round by the colorectal team.

The patient complains of a 1-day history of cough productive of purulent sputum. Nursing staff have noted that he has become increasingly short of breath over the past 48 hours and that his mobility has reduced. The team note that the patient has spiked a temperature of 38.2 degrees Celsius earlier that morning.

On examination, there is reduced air entry in the right base.

A chest X-ray confirms patchy consolidation in the right lower lobe. After sending off blood and sputum cultures, the patient is placed on empirical antibiotics.

After two days, the team is contacted by the duty microbiologist who informs them that cultures have grown *Pseudomonas Aeruginosa*.

Which of the following antibiotics are LEAST effective against this micro-organism?

A. Tazocin
B. Ceftazidime
C. Meropenem
D. Tobramycin
E. Ertapenem

36) A 58-year old man presents to the emergency department with a short history of shortness of breath, dry cough, malaise and myalgia. This has affected his ability to carry out his routine work as a farmer.

On examination, the patient is dyspnoeic at rest, he has rigors and is pyrexic with a temperature of 37.9 degrees Celsius. On auscultation of the chest, there are bi-basal fine inspiratory crackles.

Which of the following is the most likely diagnosis?

A. Cryptogenic fibrosing alveolitis
B. Extrinsic allergic alveolitis
C. Allergic bronchopulmonary aspergillosis
D. Young's syndrome
E. Byssinosis

37) A 38-year old gentleman is referred to the chest clinic due to poorly controlled asthma symptoms. He was diagnosed with asthma at the age of 32 and despite regular seretide 500 and PRN ventolin. He has ongoing shortness of breath limiting his activities of daily living. He also reports that, 2 months ago, he developed persistent numbness affecting the dorsum of his right foot.

On examination, there is marked scattered expiratory wheeze bilaterally, reduced sensation over the right foot and left palm and evidence of muscle wasting affecting the left thenar eminence.

Investigations reveal the following:

Haemoglobin	13.8g/dl	(11.5-14.0)
Mean Corpuscular Volume (MCV)	85.0fl	(82-95)
White Cell Count	12.4 x10⁹/l	(4-12)
Neutrophils	8.0 x10⁹/l	(1.2-7)
Monocytes	0.28 x10⁹/l	(0.2-0.8)
Eosinophils	1.82 x10⁹/l	(0.04-0.4)
Basophils	0.10 x10⁹/l	(0.01-0.1)

Chest X-ray report: The heart is of normal size. There is no focal lung lesion and the costophrenic angles are clear.

Which of the following is the most likely diagnosis?

A. Atopic asthma
B. Microscopic polyangiitis
C. Churg-Strauss syndrome
D. Young's syndrome
E. Wegener's granulomatosis

38) You are the junior doctor on-call and your registrar has asked you to perform an arterial blood gas on one of your patients, which reveals the following:

FiO_2	0.21	
pH	7.52	(7.35-7.45)
PaO_2	14.20 kPa	(10-13)
$PaCO_2$	2.40kPa	(4.2-6)
HCO_3^-	14.20 mEq/l	(22-28)

Which of the following is consistent with this arterial blood gas?

A. Metabolic acidosis with respiratory compensation
B. Metabolic alkalosis with respiratory compensation
C. Respiratory alkalosis with metabolic compensation
D. Respiratory acidosis with metabolic compensation
E. Mixed metabolic and respiratory alkalosis

39) You review a 58-year old male patient in the intensive care unit. On reading through the patient's notes, you find that he was admitted to hospital 7 days previously with acute onset shortness of breath.

His arterial blood gas on admission was as follows:

FiO_2	0.60	
pH	7.38	(7.35-7.45)
PaO_2	7.82 kPa	(10-13)
$PaCO_2$	5.20 kPa	(4.2-6)
HCO_3^-	22.35 mEq/l	(22-28)

Chest X-ray on admission = bilateral patchy infiltrates

Pulmonary capillary wedge pressure = 18mmHg (2-15)

Which of the following was the most likely cause for his dyspnoea?

A.   Acute left ventricular failure
B.   Acute lung injury
C.   Acute respiratory distress syndrome
D.   Pulmonary embolism
E.   Primary pulmonary hypertension

40) A 76-year old male presents to his GP with deteriorating shortness
of breath. He tells you that he previously worked as a coal miner,
but retired nearly 15 years ago. He has a 40-pack year history of
smoking.

Spirometry reveals the following:

FEV1   1.2L (predicted 2.5)
FVC   2.4L (predicted 3.0)

What is the most likely diagnosis?

A.   Simple pneumoconiosis
B.   Idiopathic pulmonary fibrosis
C.   Asbestosis
D.   Sarcoidosis
E.   Chronic obstructive pulmonary disease

Respiratory Answers

1) E: Clarithromycin

The patient's symptoms, recent holiday travel and stay at a hotel, chest X ray findings, hyponatraemia and deranged LFTs all point towards a diagnosis of Legionnaires disease; an atypical pneumonia caused by the bacterium Legionella Pneumophila. Infection with this bacterium is frequently secondary to contact with contaminated water droplets from large central air conditioning systems, humidifiers, hot water systems and cooling towers amongst other sources. It is most appropriately treated with a macrolide (clarithromycin in this case) as first line. The diagnosis can be confirmed by a positive Legionella urine antigen test. The holiday destination whereby travellers contract Legionnaires is classically quoted as Spain in exams.

2) C: Mycoplasma pneumoniae

Mycoplasma pneumoniae, Legionella pneumophila and Chlamydophila pneumoniae all cause an atypical pneumonia, best treated with macrolide antibiotics (e.g. clarithromycin, azithromycin or erythromycin). Mycoplasma pneumoniae is classically associated with cold auto-immune haemolytic anaemia, whereby antibodies produced best clump with erythrocytes at cold temperatures. This explains the positive cold agglutinin test. The haemolysis results in the formation of schistocytes, which represent sheared erythrocytes.

Additional investigations in patients with haemolytic anaemia characteristically yield an unconjugated hyperbilirubinaemia (raised indirect bilirubin), raised LDH and low haptoglobin levels. Mycoplasma can also be associated with erythema nodosum (causing painful shins), and multiple other conditions including Guillian-Barre syndrome, transverse myelitis, arthritis, endocarditis, myocarditis and rarely pancreatitis.

3) B: Aspirate with a 16-18 G cannula

This patient is haemodynamically stable and therefore is likely to have a simple, as opposed to a tension, pneumothorax. Simple spontaneous pneumothoraces can be further subdivided into primary and secondary.

According to BTS guidelines, patients are classified as having a secondary pneumothorax if they are over 50 years of age, have a significant smoking history or if there is evidence of underlying lung disease (e.g. COPD). The patient in this scenario therefore has a primary pneumothorax who, if breathless and/or a rim of >2cm is evident on the Chest X-ray, should be managed by aspiration (20-22G cannulas are too small). If the initial aspiration attempt fails, a chest drain should subsequently be inserted. Patients with secondary pneumothoraces, however, should be managed by inserting a chest drain (in the 5th intercostal space, mid-axillary line) unless the rim of air on the Chest X-ray is 1-2cm and the patient is not breathless, in which case aspiration would be appropriate.

British Thoracic Society. BTS Pleural Disease Guideline 2010.

4) **A: 0**

The CURB-65 score can be a useful and succinct method of stratifying the severity of pneumonia.

Confusion	= 1 point
Urea > 7mmol/l	= 1 point
Respiratory rate >30	= 1 point
Blood pressure (systolic <90 or diastolic <60 mmHg)	= 1 point
Age >=65	= 1 point

The following represents the 28-day mortality risks associated with the CURB scores of:

0 = 0%
1 = 1.6%
2 = 4.1%
3 = 4.9%
4 = 18.1%
5 = 28.0%

As a general rule of thumb, patients with CURB scores of 0-1 should be treated as an outpatient, 2-3 should be treated as a short stay in hospital and 4-5 requires hospitalisation with consideration of escalating care to ICU. However, the CURB scoring system should be taken with a pinch of salt and the level of treatment should be tailored according to each clinical scenario. Although the patient's CURB score is 0 in this example, nonetheless she is still likely to require admission to hospital with intravenous antibiotics and fluid resuscitation given her high respiratory rate, pyrexia and tachycardia.

Howell MD, Donnino MW, Talmor D, Clardy P, Ngo L and Shapiro NI. Performance of severity of illness scoring systems in emergency department patients with infection. Academic Emergency Medicine 14(8):709-14.

5) A: Klebsiella pneumonia

Klebsiella pneumonia has a tendency to affect immunocompromised hosts (e.g. elderly, diabetics and alcoholics), with a predilection for the upper lobes. It can cause a cavitating pneumonia, like staphylococcus aureus (which classically occurs after influenza infection) and mycobacteria tuberculosis. However, cavitating lesions occur in secondary, not primary tuberculosis. Additionally, the history is too short to represent a typical case of secondary tuberculosis. Mycoplasma pneumonia produces an insidious illness, often lasting more than a week, with a progressive dry cough and constitutional upset with headaches, myalgia and rash (e.g. erythema nodosum or erythema multiforme).

6) E: Chronic obstructive pulmonary disease

Clubbing occurs in stages. First there is softening and increased fluctuance of the nail bed. Next, there is loss of the Lovibond angle (loss of the normal <165 degree angle between the nail plate and the proximal nailfold), followed by increased curvature of the nail plate. Finally, there is expansion of the terminal phalanx giving the so-called 'drumsticking' appearance. Other respiratory causes of clubbing include lung abscess, empyema and lung cancer (in particular, squamous cell carcinoma of the lung). Clubbing in a patient with COPD should raise the question of a possible undiagnosed lung malignancy (as smoking is a risk factor for both aetiologies) or other possible non-respiratory causes of clubbing.

7) **D: 30-49%**

FEV1 represents the forced expiratory volume over 1 second and can be measured by spirometry. FEV1% predicted refers to the FEV1 value as a percentage of that predicted when compared with a healthy individual without COPD, controlling for age, sex and height measurements. Mild, moderate, severe and very severe COPD correspond to the FEV1% predicted values of ≥ 80%, 50-79%, 30-49% and < 30%, respectively.

8) **D: Tiotropium inhaler**

According to NICE guidelines, COPD patients with symptoms inadequately controlled by a short-acting beta-2 agonist (SABA) or short-acting muscarinic antagonist (SAMA) as required should have their FEV1 assessed, as this will dictate further management. If their FEV1 is ≥50% predicted, as in this example, then the next option is to supplement their current pharmacological regimen (PRN SABA/SAMA) with either a long acting beta-2 agonist (LABA) such as salmeterol or a long-acting muscarinic antagonist (LAMA) (i.e. tiotropium). If the FEV1 is < 50% predicted, then the PRN SABA/SAMA should be supplemented with either a LABA + inhaled corticosteroid combination inhaler (ICS) such as seretide (salmeterol and fluticasone) or LAMA. If these options fail to control the patient's COPD, then a combination of LAMA + LABA + ICS may be tried.

Seretide 250 and 500 correspond to a dose of 250 and 500 micrograms of fluticasone, respectively, per blister in the accuhaler.

National Institute for Health and Clinical Excellence 2010. Chronic obstructive pulmonary disease. CG 101. London: National Institute for Health and Clinical Excellence.

9) E: Oxygen Saturations 94%

Options A to D are all features of acute severe asthma. The features of acute life-threatening asthma, which demands more urgent treatment, a lower threshold for escalation of care to ITU and earlier consideration for pre-emptive intubation and ventilation, are shown below:

a) $SpO_2 < 92\%$
b) Peak expiratory flow (PEF) < 33% best or predicted
c) $PaO_2 < 8kPa$
d) Normal or raised $PaCO_2$
e) Cyanosis
f) Arrhythmia
g) Silent chest, poor respiratory effort or exhaustion

Note that as patients with acute asthma attacks often hyperventilate, a reduced $PaCO_2$ would be expected on an arterial blood gas. If patients become exhausted and enter a life-threatening phase, however, respiratory depression ensues, causing CO_2 levels to rise to within or even above the normal range.

The British Thoracic Society, Scottish Intercollegiate Guidelines Network. British Guidelines on the Management of Asthma. *May 2011.*

10) A: IV Magnesium 1.2-2g over 20 minutes

Acute severe and life-threatening asthma exacerbations are medical emergencies. Patients should be sat up, given 100% oxygen via a non-rebreathing bag, salbutamol (2.5-5mg) and ipratropium (500 micrograms) via oxygen-driven nebulisers, which can be repeated at 10-15 minute intervals, and intravenous hydrocortisone (100mg stat dose). If these measures fail, then IV magnesium sulphate 1.2-2g over 20 minutes should be considered with a view to calling for senior support and ITU if necessary. Salbutamol is very rarely given intravenously and should only be considered by someone senior who is experienced in its use.

The British Thoracic Society, Scottish Intercollegiate Guidelines Network. British Guidelines on the Management of Asthma. *May 2011.*

11) C: Trial of non-invasive ventilation

This patient has an exacerbation of COPD, for which he is receiving optimal medical therapy. The ABG shows evidence of type II respiratory failure (defined as a $PaO_2 < 8kPa$ and $PaCO_2 > 6kPa$), i.e. 'he is retaining CO_2.' Although lowering the inspired oxygen concentration to 24% may begin to correct the hypercapnia, his already significant hypoxia will worsen. According to BTS guidelines, COPD patients who remain in type II respiratory failure despite optimal medical therapy should receive a trial of non-invasive ventilation (NIV) providing that there is evidence of persistent respiratory acidosis (pH<7.35, $PaCO_2$ >6.0kPa) on the ABG. Intubation and ventilation should only be considered after NIV has failed, or if the patient is in extremis and NIV would be an inappropriate intermediary step. Given this patient's age and multiple co-morbidities, it is unlikely that he will be an appropriate candidate for intubation and ventilation.

Concise Guidance to Good Practise. Non-invasive ventilation in chronic obstructive pulmonary disease: management of acute type 2 respiratory failure. National Guidelines. 2008.

12) D: Serum ACE is raised in approximately 20% of patients

The constellation of symptoms, clinical signs and investigation findings make a diagnosis of sarcoidosis most likely. Sarcoidosis is a chronic, non-caseating granulomatous disorder of uncertain aetiology that can potentially affect any organ system. The reported prevalence varies according to age (incidence peaks at 20-39 years of age), sex (slightly commoner in women), geographical location (more frequent in northern European countries), and ethnicity (3 times commoner in African-Americans than white Americans). In the UK, the incidence is approximately 10-20 per 100,000 of the population.

Sarcoidosis most commonly affects the lungs (>90% cases) with patients often presenting with an insidious history of progressive breathlessness, dry cough and lethargy. Examination of the lungs is often unremarkable; crackles may be heard in advanced disease when pulmonary fibrosis predominates with a predilection for the upper lobes. Although bilateral hilar lymphadenopathy is the classically described radiological finding of sarcoidosis, it is not pathognomonic of the condition as it can also occur in tuberculosis and lymphoma.

Pulmonary sarcoidosis can progress in stages with an increasingly poor prognosis:

Stage 1 =   bi-hilar lymphadenopathy only.

Stage 2 =   bi-hilar lymphadenopathy plus pulmonary infiltrates.

Stage 3 =   pulmonary infiltrates only

Stage 4 =   pulmonary fibrosis

Other clinical manifestations include:

a)   Fatigue (66%)
b)   Dermatological (24%) = erythema nodosum (a panniculitis characterised by tender red nodules commonly affecting the shins) and lupus pernio (as in this example)
c)   Lymphadenopathy (15%)
d)   Ocular involvement (12%) = anterior and/or posterior uveitis (this patient has an anterior uveitis with synechia accounting for the irregularly shaped pupil), lacrimal gland enlargement and optic neuropathy.
e)   Renal (5%) = extra-renal macrophages in sarcoid granulomas can produce 1-alpha hydroxylase, which increases the production of 1,25 dihydroxycholecalciferol, causing a hypercalcaemia in 11% of patients. Renal calculi develop in 10% of patients with sarcoidosis.
f)   Neurological (5%) = the facial nerve is most commonly affected, but an aseptic meningitis and encephalopathy can also rarely occur
g)   Cardiac (2%)
h)   Musculoskeletal (0.9%) = arthralgia being the most common

A classical investigation, though not commonly performed nowadays, may be asked in exams. This is the Kveim-Siltzbach test, which involves intra-dermally injecting homogenised human sarcoid tissue into a patient suspected of having sarcoidosis, and then taking a biopsy of the injection site after 4-weeks. The test is positive if new sarcoid granulomas have formed.

The correct answer is D as serum ACE is raised in approximately 60% of patients with sarcoidosis.

Dempsey OJ, Paterson EW, Kerr KM, Denison AR. Sarcoidosis. British Medical Journal. 2009;339: 620-25.

13) E: Asbestosis

Pulmonary fibrosis in asbestosis and rheumatoid arthritis preferentially involves the lower lobes. Remember the mnemonic: TEARS: TB, Extrinsic Allergic Alveolitis, Ankylosing Spondylitis, Radiotherapy, Sarcoidosis – as causes of upper lobe fibrosis.

14) E: A 28-year old male found to have bilateral hilar lymphadenopathy and pulmonary infiltrates on the chest X –ray

Hypercalcemia, neurological, cardiac and ocular involvement (refractory to topical steroid therapy) in sarcoidosis all represent absolute indications for oral steroid therapy. Patients with stable stage 2 or 3 disease (stage 2 in this example) is not an absolute indication for oral steroids providing that lung function is only mildly impaired.

UK guidelines recommend initial treatment with 0.5mg/kg/day of prednisolone for 4 weeks, the dose of which is then gradually tapered to a maintenance dose of 10mg or less/day. Duration of steroid treatment for sarcoidosis is often 6-24 months at least.

Dempsey OJ, Paterson EW, Kerr KM, Denison AR. Sarcoidosis. British Medical Journal. 2009;339: 620-25.

15) C: Stop salmeterol and increase beclomethasone to 800 micrograms/day

The management of asthma has been divided into 5 steps according to BTS guidelines:

Step 1 *(mild intermittent asthma)*
PRN inhaled short-acting beta-2 agonist (SABA), e.g. salbutamol

Step 2 *(regular preventer therapy)*
Add inhaled steroid 200-800 micrograms per day, the exact dose being titrated according to the severity of disease

Step 3 *(initial add-on therapy)*
Add inhaled long-acting beta-2 agonist (LABA), like salmeterol.
- If there is a good response to this treatment, continue LABA.
- If benefit is derived from LABA but asthma control remains inadequate, continue treatment but also increase inhaled steroid to 800 micrograms/day.
- If there is no benefit from LABA (as in this scenario), stop LABA and increase inhaled steroid to 800 micrograms/day

Step 4 *(persistent poor control)*
- Increase inhaled steroid to 2000 micrograms/day
- Addition of leukotriene receptor antagonist (e.g. Monteleukast), SR theophylline or beta-2 agonist tablet

Step 5 *(continuous or frequent use of oral steroids)*

Commence oral steroid therapy, refer patient for specialist care and always consider other treatments to minimise the use of oral steroids.

The British Thoracic Society, Scottish Intercollegiate Guidelines Network. British Guidelines on the Management of Asthma. May 2011.

16) C: Squamous cell lung carcinoma

Lung cancer is the second most common cancer and the most common cause of cancer-related deaths in the UK. It is generally divided into small cell (18% of lung cancer) and non-small cell lung cancers (78%). Non-small cell lung cancers can be further subdivided into squamous cell, adenocarcinoma and large cell carcinoma. Cigarette smoking remains the single biggest risk factor for the development of lung cancer.

Out of all lung cancers, squamous cell carcinoma is the most common subtype and is the one that is most frequently associated with hypercalcaemia. This often arises due to the production of parathyroid hormone (PTH)-related peptide by the neoplastic cells, which stimulates calcium reabsorption from the distal renal tubules.

http://www.cancerresearchuk.org/cancer-help/type/lung-cancer/about/ types-of-lung-cancer

17) **D: Small cell lung carcinoma**

It is clear that this patient is very likely to have some form of lung malignancy. He is at high risk because of his age, smoking history and the presence of other red flag features including weight loss and loss of appetite. The chest X-ray confirms the presence of a suspicious lung lesion (mesothelioma would appear as diffuse, irregular pleural thickening with or without pleural effusion).

The results of his investigations show that this patient has a syndrome of inappropriate ADH (SIADH) release, which in this case scenario represents a paraneoplastic phenomenon. Recall that SIADH is a common cause of hyponatraemia, but is a diagnosis of exclusion.

The following criteria must be met for a diagnosis of SIADH to be made:

a)   Hyponatraemia
b)   Inappropriately concentrated urine (> 100mOsm/kg, but is often higher than serum osmolality)
c)   Urinary natriuresis > 40mmol/l
d)   Normal renal, adrenal, thyroid, cardiac and liver function (as failure of any of these organs can cause hyponatraemia)
e)   Euvolaemic on examination

Answering this question correctly requires the knowledge that of all lung cancers, small cell lung carcinoma (SCLC) is most commonly associated with SIADH (15-40% of SCLC patients develop SIADH).

Other paraneoplastic syndromes classically associated with SCLC include:

a) *Cushing's syndrome* (2-5% of SCLC patients)
b) *Lambert-Eaton syndrome* (This is caused by the production of auto-antibodies that target voltage-gated calcium channels in the pre-synaptic nerve terminals of neuromuscular junctions. Patients develop a proximally distributed muscle weakness most pronounced in the lower limbs. Improvement in reflex activity after muscle contraction and facilitation of muscle action potential amplitudes during repetitive stimulation on EMG testing are characteristic hallmarks of Lambert-Eaton syndrome. Although only 2-5% of SCLC patients develop this syndrome, 50% of patients with Lambert-Eaton syndrome have or develop SCLC).

SCLC constitute 18% of all lung cancers in the UK. They generally have a central location on chest radiographs, have a tendency for early dissemination and are often highly sensitive to chemotherapy. Despite good initial response to chemotherapy, patients often relapse and the prognosis remains poor with a 5-year survival rate of less than 5%.

Cancer research UK. http://www.cancerresearchuk.org/cancer-help/type/lung-cancer/treatment/statistics-and-outlook-for-lung-cancer#small

Van Meerbeeck JP, Fennell DA and De Ruysscher DKM. Small-cell lung cancer. The Lancet. 2011;378: 1741-55

Decaux G and Musch W. Clinical laboratory evaluation of the syndrome of inappropriate secretion of antidiuretic hormone. Clinical Journal of the American Society of Nephrology. 2008;3:1175-84.

18) E: Nephrotic syndrome

The patient has a right-sided pleural effusion (note that although pleural effusions are classically described as 'stony dull' to percussion on chest examination, it is very difficult to clinically differentiate between 'dull' and 'stony dull').

The investigation findings suggest that the effusion is exudative (i.e. protein-rich), meaning that nephrotic syndrome, which causes a transudative effusion, is the least likely diagnosis.

Pleural fluid with protein >35g/L is an exudate, whilst pleural fluid with protein < 25g/L is a transudate (in reality, it's not always clear cut).

Light's criteria can also be used to differentiate between exudates and transudates. An effusion is an exudate if at least one of the following is present:

a) Pleural fluid: serum protein > 0.5
b) Pleural fluid: serum LDH > 0.6
c) Pleural fluid LDH > 2/3 upper limit of normal serum LDH

An alternative method of differentiating pleural exudates from transudates is to calculate the serum to pleural albumin gradient by subtracting pleural albumin from serum albumin. A value of less than 12 g/L is consistent with an exudate.

The causes of exudates include:

a) Empyema
b) Pneumonia
c) Lung malignancy
d) Tuberculosis
e) Rheumatoid arthritis
f) Pulmonary embolism
g) Systemic lupus erythematosus (SLE)

Causes of transudates include:

a)   Heart failure
b)   Liver failure
c)   Chronic renal failure
d)   Nephrotic syndrome
e)   Hypoalbuminaemia
f)   Pulmonary embolism (but more commonly causes exudates)

Light RW, MacGregor I, Luchsinger PC and Ball WC. Pleural Effusions: The Diagnostic Separation of Transudates and Exudates. Annals of Internal Medicine. 1972;77:507-13.

Light, RW. Pleural effusion due to pulmonary emboli. Current Opinion in Pulmonary Medicine. 2001; 7:198-201

19) B: Asbestosis

Given this patient's occupational history he is likely to have been exposed to asbestos. The use of asbestos was ubiquitous in the 19th and 20th centuries owing to its many attractive properties; it has high tensile strength and is resistant to multiple forms of destruction including heat, fire, electrical and chemical damage. The fibrous nature of asbestos allows it to be easily woven into cement materials, ceiling tiles, pipe and boiler insulation, flooring, brakes and clutch linings, polymers and resins.

Patients who are likely to have had heavy exposure to asbestos may have previously had or worked in any number of occupations, including asbestos miners, builders, electricians, plumbers, workers in the shipyard or car manufacturing industry. The use of asbestos had later declined owing to the discoveries of its significant adverse effects on the lungs and pleura.

Asbestosis is an example of pneumoconiosis, which is defined as an interstitial lung disease caused by the inhalation of inorganic dusts, in this case asbestos. This ultimately leads to pulmonary fibrosis, a restrictive lung disease causing progressive dyspnoea and hypoxaemia. Typical examination findings are finger clubbing and bi-basal fine inspiratory crackles.

The patient's previous occupation points us towards a diagnosis of asbestosis. Silicosis, berylliosis and siderosis are all interstitial lung diseases that can produce the same clinical features as asbestosis, but arise due to previous heavy exposure to silica, beryllium and iron dusts, respectively. Silicosis classically occurs in sandblasters, berylliosis in aerospace industry workers and siderosis in iron ore miners. Idiopathic Pulmonary Fibrosis (also known as cryptogenic fibrosing alveolitis) would have been correct had the cause been unknown.

Other asbestos-related lung diseases include lung cancer, which has a multiplicative interaction with cigarette smoking, and malignant mesothelioma. Patients with malignant mesothelioma can present with chest pain, which if often dull, diffuse and progressive, though occasionally pleuritic, along with red flag features such as anorexia, weight loss and importantly, a history of asbestos exposure, which dramatically raises the risk.

Different types of asbestos exist including the serpentine fibrous type (chrysotile; white asbestos) or amphibole straight fibres (crocidolite (blue), amosite (brown) and anthophyllite). Blue and brown asbestos are, relatively speaking, often considered the most dangerous subtypes.

Completely benign and often asymptomatic asbestos-related lung disease include pleural plaques and diffuse pleural thickening, though the latter can also occur secondary to tuberculosis, previous haemothorax, chest surgery, drug (e.g. methysergide) and radiation exposure. Although benign pleural effusions can also occur secondary to previous asbestos exposure, this is a diagnosis of exclusion as many other causes of pleural effusion must be considered first, including malignant mesothelioma.

Currie GP, Watt SJ and Maskell NA. An overview of how asbestos exposure affects the lung. British Medical Journal. 2009;339: 506-10.

20) E: 20-35 years

Because of the long latency period between asbestos exposure and corresponding lung/pleural disease, it is always important to take a detailed occupational history from a patient presenting with respiratory disease.

Currie GP, Watt SJ and Maskell NA. An overview of how asbestos exposure affects the lung. British Medical Journal. 2009;339: 506-10.

21) B: Partial pressure of oxygen dissolved in arterial plasma

The PaO_2 is the partial pressure of oxygen dissolved in arterial plasma (whereas the PAO_2 is the partial pressure of oxygen in the alveoli); it gives no indication as to how much oxygen is combined with haemoglobin. Remember that when interpreting arterial blood gases, it is imperative to state the FiO_2 (fraction of inspired oxygen). A PaO_2 of 14 kPa is perfectly normal for a healthy patient breathing room air (21% oxygen, i.e. FiO_2 of 0.21), whilst the same PaO_2 value in someone breathing high flow oxygen via a non-rebreathing mask would be considered pathologically low.

22) E: A 24-year old lady on the combined oral contraceptive pill

Risk factors for deep vein thrombosis (DVT) and pulmonary embolism (PE) can be divided into major and minor risk factors:

Major risk factors (relative risk increased 5-20 fold) include:

a) Recent lower limb orthopaedic surgery
b) Recent major and/or abdominal surgery
c) Malignancy – pelvic, abdominal, metastatic disease
d) Fractures, varicose veins, reduced mobility of any cause
e) Previous DVT or PE
f) Obstetrics – late pregnancy (third trimester), pre-eclampsia

Minor risk factors (relative risk increased 2-4 fold) include:

a) Oestrogens – hormone replacement therapy (HRT), oral contraceptives (particularly third generation pills)
b) Cardiovascular – congenital heart disease, heart failure, hypertension
c) Other – occult malignancy, obesity, nephrotic syndrome, inflammatory bowel disease

Robinson G. Pulmonary embolism: an update on diagnosis and management. 2012. BMJ learning.

23) D: Give 120mg enoxaparin, arrange a CTPA and, if positive, continue daily 120mg enoxaparin lifelong

Given that this patient has metastatic malignancy, she is at high risk of thromboembolic events. In this case, the sudden onset worsening of dyspnoea and tachypnoea (respiratory rate> 20) means that she is likely to have had a pulmonary embolism (PE). The diagnosis is further supported by her desaturation and by her Arterial Blood Gas (ABG), which shows type 1 respiratory failure. Note that in a PE, the mechanism of hypoxaemia is a ventilation/perfusion (V/Q) mismatch, as the clot causes certain areas of affected lung tissue that are ventilated to no longer receive perfusion. The low $PaCO_2$ in this example is secondary to hyperventilation. For a given PaO_2, the prognosis is poorer the lower the $PaCO_2$. This is because it implies a higher rate of ventilation is only enough to produce a PaO_2 of the same level, meaning that the V/Q mismatch is of greater severity.

Acute PE can present in multiple different ways, as follows:

a) *Pulmonary infarction syndrome (60%):* patients characteristically present with sudden onset pleuritic chest pain (well-localised pain described as sharp/stabbing in nature and exacerbated by inspiration), which may be accompanied by haemoptysis. Sudden shortness of breath is a commonly associated feature. Infarcted lung can classically appear as a wedge of opacification on a chest X-ray, which may be accompanied by a pleural effusion (small effusions being present in 40% of patients).

b) *Isolated dyspnoea (25%):* As in this example, patients with PE may present with only sudden onset shortness of breath and tachypnoea without any chest pain or circulatory compromise.

c) *Collapse, poor reserve (10%):* This presentation can occur in elderly patients where a loss of consciousness is the sole presenting feature of a PE.

d) *Haemodynamic collapse in a previously well patient (5%):* This is where the previously fit and well patient presents with shock. This clinical presentation may arise due to a massive PE (i.e. saddle PE), which causes acute right heart strain and significant haemodynamic compromise. Right heart strain on a 12-lead ECG may appear as a right bundle branch block (RBBB), T-wave inversion in the anterior precordial leads (V1-V4) and/or right axis deviation (other ECG features in PE include sinus tachycardia – most common, AF and the classical, but rare S1Q3T3 pattern). Patients with massive PE and significant haemodynamic compromise or shock, may qualify for thrombolysis. An urgent inpatient echocardiogram is recommended in such patients to assess the degree of cardiac compromise.

Patients may also present with a chronic PE-type picture with insidious breathlessness over a period of weeks to months.

Examination findings

This may be unremarkable. However the following can be seen:

1) Tachypnoea
2) Atrial fibrillation (AF)
3) Tachycardia; most commonly this is sinus tachycardia, but may also be due to fast AF
4) Pleural rub or signs of a pleural effusion, often seen in pulmonary infarction syndrome
5) Signs of right heart failure (e.g. raised JVP, hepatomegaly, pedal oedema)
6) Signs of a DVT (swelling of the leg/calf, calf tenderness, erythema) in 25% of patients with PE
7) Loud P2 and splitting of the second heart sound

Treatment

Anyone for whom there is a strong clinical suspicion of PE should receive treatment-dose clexane (enoxaparin) (1.5 mg/kg subcutaneously, once daily) without delay, providing there are no contra-indications. Treatment-dose clexane should be differentiated from the lower prophylactic dose; the latter is given to prevent the development of thromboembolic disease as opposed to treating it.

If further investigations, namely a V/Q scan or CTPA as in this example, exclude the presence of a PE, then treatment-dose clexane can either be stopped or switched back to prophylactic dose depending on the clinical situation. If a pulmonary embolism is confirmed, however, then under normal circumstances the patient can be considered for warfarin (6 months duration for a single event) with a target INR of 2-3. Option C would have been correct if the patient did not have a history of metastatic malignancy.

Avoiding anticoagulation with warfarin, and giving lifelong clexane is the preferred option in patients with advanced malignancy and confirmed DVT/PE. Life-long clexane is also preferred in patients who are deemed unsuitable for warfarin treatment for many other reasons, including instances where there are difficulties in monitoring the patient's INR or the patient is deemed unable to comply with warfarin due to cognitive impairment for example.

Robinson G. Pulmonary embolism: an update on diagnosis and management. 2012. BMJ learning.

British Thoracic Society guidelines for the management of acute pulmonary embolism. Thorax 2003;58:470-84.

24) A: Pulmonary arteriography

This is a trick question. Although rarely performed in clinical practice, pulmonary arteriography, which is a highly invasive procedure that involves right heart and direct pulmonary artery catheterization, is described as the gold-standard investigation for PE. CTPA and V/Q scans are performed far, far more commonly in clinical practice. Doppler USS is used to investigate DVT, not PE.

Whenever investigating a patient for a PE, it is always important to calculate an estimate of the patient's pre-test probability score. In other words, try to stratify the patient's chances of having had a PE before undertaking any tests or investigations. This can be done by considering the following:

a) Patients must have clinical features compatible with a PE, i.e. dyspnoea, tachypnoea, pleuritic chest pain, haemoptysis etc.

b) There is no alternative explanation for the patient's symptoms. For example, if the patient is dyspnoeic, but he/she is also pyrexic and there is consolidation on a chest X-ray, then pneumonia can explain the patient's symptoms. If there is no alternative explanation for the patient's symptoms, then this makes the diagnosis of a PE more likely.

c) There is a major risk factor, which predisposes the patient to a PE (see previous question)

The pre-test probability of PE is:

1) Low if only a) is fulfilled
2) Intermediate if a) and, b) or c) are fulfilled
3) High if a), b) and c) are fulfilled

Note that a similar scoring system can equally be adapted to DVT.

A D-dimer is a sensitive, but not specific test for thromboembolic disease, as it is invariably raised in many conditions as well as in thromboembolism. For example, any inflammatory condition, trauma, prolonged bed rest, even old age, can all raise D-Dimer levels.

A D-dimer is useful only if it is negative because, with a low pre-test probability and negative D-dimer result, there is a 90% chance of definitively excluding a DVT or PE.

Anyone for whom there is a strong clinical suspicion of DVT/PE (intermediate/high pre-test probability) should automatically be considered for a Doppler USS (in suspected DVT) or a CTPA or V/Q scan (in suspected PE).

British Thoracic Society guidelines for the management of acute pulmonary embolism. Thorax 2003;58:470-84.

Robinson G. Pulmonary embolism: an update on diagnosis and management. 2012. BMJ learning.

25) B: IV pentamidine

This patient has pneumocystis jiroveci pneumonia (formerly called pneumocystis carinii), an infection in which immunocompromised patients with a CD4 T cell count of less than 200 cells/mm^3 are highly susceptible to developing. Not only are HIV positive patients with acquired immunodeficiency syndrome (AIDS) at risk, but all immunocompromised patients are, including those on high dose steroids for protracted time periods, those on chemotherapy and post-transplant patients whom invariably receive a cocktail of immunosuppressant drugs.

Patients with pneumocystis jiroveci pneumonia commonly present with a several weeks- history of progressive dyspnoea, dry cough, fever and difficulty taking in a deep breath. Clinical examination often reveals tachypnoea, tachycardia, and sometimes cyanosis. Auscultation of the chest is commonly unremarkable, but there may be evidence of scattered crackles bilaterally. A characteristic feature of pneumocystis jiroveci pneumonia is that patients often desaturate markedly on relatively minimal exertion as is evident in this example. Chest radiography typically shows perihilar or diffuse interstitial infiltrates with ground-glass shadowing but may be normal in at least one third of cases. Less common features include lobar consolidation, pleural effusions and cavitating lesions.

The gold standard investigation for pneumocystis jiroveci is open lung biopsy, though this is rarely performed in clinical practice. Less invasive procedures like bronchoalveolar lavage during bronchoscopy and sputum induction are commonly employed methods.

First line treatment for pneumocystis jiroveci pneumonia is high dose co-trimoxazole (septrin), which is a combination of trimethoprim and sulphamethoxazole (a sulphonamide) that act synergistically, and sequentially inhibit two enzymes involved in folate metabolism. As this patient is allergic to trimethoprim, the correct answer is IV pentamidine, which represents an alternative treatment. Other drugs that can be used to treat this condition include clindamycin and oral primaquine.

Wilkin A and Feinberg. Pneumocystis carinii Pneumonia: A Clinical Review. American Family Physician. 1999;60:1699-1708

Wazir JF and Ansari NA. Pneumocystis carinii Infection. Archives of Pathology and Laboratory Medicine. 2004;128: 1023-27

26) E: Amlodipine

Pulmonary fibrosis is not a recognised side effect of amlodipine.

27) B: Bilateral basal fine late inspiratory crackles

Fine late inspiratory crackles, which sounds similar to rubbing hair between the fingers is heard in pulmonary fibrosis. These crackles occur as a result of the alveoli and small bronchioles opening up during inspiration.

Fine early to mid-inspiratory crackles are typically heard in pulmonary oedema (though not as fine as in pulmonary fibrosis!).

Coarse crackles are typically heard in bronchiectasis and pneumonia.

Douglas G, Nicol F and Robertson C. Macleod's Clinical Examination. Churchill Livingstone, Elsevier. 12ᵗʰ Edition. Page 174.

28) D: Intravenous co-amoxiclav 1.2g TDS and oral clarithromycin 500mg BD

For a diagnosis of pneumonia to be made there must be:

a) Clinical evidence of lower respiratory tract symptoms (e.g. shortness of breath/cough)
b) Evidence that such symptoms are of infective origin (e.g. mucus production, more purulent mucus, temperature spikes, rising inflammatory markers) AND
c) Radiological evidence of consolidation.

This patient has a CURB-65 score of 4 and therefore has pneumonia of high severity.
According to BTS guidelines, patients with pneumonia of the following severities should be treated with the antibiotic regimens as shown below:

Low severity (CURB-65 score 0-1) = oral amoxicillin 500mg TDS (three times daily).

Moderate severity (CURB-65 score 2) = oral amoxicillin 500mg-1g
TDS and oral clarithromycin 500mg BD (twice daily)
High severity (CURB-65 score 3-5) = intravenous co-amoxiclav 1.2g
TDS and oral clarithromycin 500mg BD

Penicillin-allergic patients with low or moderately severe pneumonia
can be treated with oral doxycycline (200mg loading dose followed by
100mg BD). Alternative agents include levofloxacin or a combination
of vancomycin and clarithromycin for severe pneumonia.

Note that the type of antibiotics recommended as first line treatment
will vary according to local microbial resistance patterns and local
prescribing policies.

*British Thoracic Society. Guidelines for the management of community
acquired pneumonia in adults. Thorax. 2009.*

29) D: pH 7.35, PaO$_2$ 6.8, PaCO$_2$ 8.4, HCO$_3$ 33.61

Option D is the correct answer. The definition of type II respiratory
failure is a PaO$_2$ < 8kPa combined with a PaCO$_2$ > 6kPa. Although
option E fulfils this criterion, it is incorrect because in chronic type
II respiratory failure, the kidneys would be expected to reabsorb
bicarbonate ions in an effort to buffer the pH to within the normal
range.

Option A is consistent with a severe metabolic acidosis with
attempted respiratory compensation (e.g. diabetic ketoacidosis with
Kussmaul's breathing).

Option B is consistent with type 1 respiratory failure (PaO2 < 8kPa,
but PaCO2 4.5-6kPa, i.e. normal PaCO2), e.g. seen in pulmonary
embolism/fibrosis/oedema, pneumothorax, acute severe/life-
threatening asthma and sometimes in COPD.

Option C represents respiratory alkalosis, typically seen in
psychogenic hyperventilation and salicylate poisoning.

30) A: 73-year old male with bronchiectasis and a PaO₂, which is consistently 7.4kPa on air

Multiple multicentre trials (the first two landmark studies being the MRC and NOTT trials) have repeatedly shown that long-term oxygen therapy (LTOT) can improve survival in a select group of patients with chronic respiratory/heart failure if they receive oxygen for at least 15-18 hours/day. Certain criteria need to be fulfilled before a patient can be considered for LTOT. These are:

1) Patients must have evidence of chronic hypoxaemia, despite optimal medical treatment, with a PaO2 of <7.3kPa on air, measured on separate occasions (usually at least 3 weeks apart). Or, patients can have a stable PaO2 of 7.3-8.0 kPa providing that they also have evidence of secondary polycythaemia and/or clinical/echocardiographic evidence of pulmonary hypertension

   AND

2) Absence of an exacerbation of chronic lung disease within the previous five weeks.

LTOT may also be prescribed for terminally ill patients as a palliative measure.

British Thoracic Society (January 2006). Report on Clinical Component for the Home Oxygen Service in England and Wales.

(MRC) Medical Research Council Working Party. Long term domiciliary oxygen therapy in chronic hypoxic cor pulmonale complicating chronic bronchitis and emphysema. Report of the Medical Research Council Working Party. Lancet. 1981;1:681–5.

(NOTT) Nocturnal Oxygen Therapy Trial Group. Continuous or nocturnal oxygen therapy in hypoxemic chronic obstructive lung disease: a clinical trial. Nocturnal Oxygen Therapy Trial Group. Annals of Internal Medicine. 1980;93:391–8.

31) C: Secondary Tuberculosis

Tuberculosis remains a significant global health burden with a worldwide incidence of approximately 8-10 million per year, accounting for around 1.7 million deaths each year. It is a chronic granulomatous disease caused by Mycobacteria Tuberculosis, which is an acid-fast, aerobic, non-spore forming, non-motile, non-encapsulated, obligate intracellular pathogen.

Primary tuberculosis is the pattern of disease, which develops in a person that has not previously been exposed, and is therefore un-sensitised, to the tubercle bacilli. It is asymptomatic in the majority of cases. It takes around 3 weeks for the immunocompetent host to mount an immune response to mycobacteria tuberculosis. The nature of the immune response is a CD4-positive Th1 cell mediated hypersensitivity response (type IV hypersensitivity). Activated Th1 cells release IL-2, which promotes self-proliferation, and interferon-gamma secretion, which activates macrophages to target the mycobacteria bacilli. The activated macrophages produce more cytokines, including TNF-alpha and chemokines, which induce the recruitment of more monocytes and T-cells to the focus of infection. The result is the formation of granulomas with central caseous necrosis, epithelioid cells, giant cells and monocytes walling of the infection, all collectively representing the histological hallmark of tuberculosis. Macroscopically, this focus of inflammatory response is called the Ghon focus, which is typically found in the lower part of the upper lobe or the upper part of the lower lobe. As the tubercular bacilli drain to the hilar nodes, the inflammatory process can lead to hilar lymphadenopathy. This combination of parenchymal and nodal involvement is called the Ghon complex. The Ghon complex later undergoes fibrosis and calcification with no further progression of the lesions, unless the host's immunity declines. In certain immune-compromised hosts, such as those with AIDS, or malnourished and elderly patients, the initial infection can progress and cause progressive primary tuberculosis, whose clinical manifestation closely resembles an acute bacterial pneumonia. This may lead to middle or lower lobar consolidation with hilar lymphadenopathy and pleural effusion, but not cavitation.

Secondary tuberculosis (also called post-primary TB) is the pattern of disease, which arises in a patient who has previously been sensitised to mycobacteria tuberculosis. Any time after primary tuberculosis, up to several decades after primary infection, the dormant lesions can become reactivated. The reactivated chronic granulomatous response ultimately manifests as the formation of cavitating lesions, classically affecting one or both upper lobes. Here, patients typically present with an insidious muco-purulent cough, usually of 3 or more weeks' duration, along with constitutional symptoms spanning anorexia, weight loss, fever and night sweats. Haemoptysis and pleuritic chest pain are other presenting pulmonary features. Secondary tuberculosis is often the result of a weakening of the host's level of immunity as it can occur in elderly, alcoholics, malnourished patients, patients exposed to chemotherapy and prolonged steroid use. Secondary tuberculosis is an AIDS-defining illness, explaining why all patients with clinical manifestations of tuberculosis should be offered an HIV test.

Miliary tuberculosis most often affects immunocompromised patients and represents diffuse spread of tubercular bacilli throughout the lungs (radiographic appearance suggestive of 'millet seeds' throughout the lung fields), and even systemically. TB can potentially affect any organ system including:

a) Central nervous system - manifesting as meningitis (typically insidious onset-symptoms of headache, fever, neck stiffness, vomiting), encephalitis, brain abscesses, (cranial) nerve palsies

b) Genitourinary system –may present with features of pyelonephritis such as loin pain, fever, rigors and lower urinary tract symptoms (e.g. dysuria, frequency, urgency). Infertility.

c) Skin – apple jelly nodules of lupus vulgaris (cutaneous TB)

d) Cardiovascular – constrictive pericarditis, pericardial effusion, endocarditis

e) Bone and joints – osteomyelitis, Pott's disease (spinal TB), septic arthritis

f) Hepatobiliary – liver/splenic abscesses

Any patient with suspected TB should have their sputum (or any sample including pus, CSF, urine, blood) sent for microscopy and culture. Three consecutive early morning urine and sputum samples should be sent. Microscopic diagnosis may be via smear stains (where the Tubercular bacilli are classically stained with Ziehl Neelsen stains) or via fluorescent microscopy, the latter displaying greater sensitivity. Gold standard diagnosis remains with culture (with highest yields from biopsied specimens), as it also allows drug sensitivities to be established. TB blood cultures usually require up to 6-10 weeks (e.g. in Lowenstein-Jensen media), but more recent liquid media-based assays can accelerate detection to within 2 weeks. Molecular techniques, such as PCR have aided greater rapidity of diagnosis.

The Mantoux test is a useful screening test that can be used to detect previous exposure to mycobacteria, by measuring the maximum diameter of skin induration (not erythema) 48-72 hours after intradermal injection of tuberculin antigen. The Mantoux test result can be graded as follows:

a) Less than 5 mm induration; test is negative = no previous exposure to Mycobacteria Tuberculosis, patients can receive the BCG vaccination
b) 5-15mm induration; positive test = indicates hypersensitivity to tuberculin; this may be due to previous BCG vaccination, previous exposure to TB or other atypical mycobacteria (e.g. M. avium intraclulare, M. Bovis etc)
c) Greater than 15mm induration; strongly positive = usually suggestive of TB infection (atypical mycobacteria often result in smaller areas of induration)

However, the Mantoux test is subject to false positives (e.g. atypical mycobacterial infection, previous BCG vaccination) and false negatives (e.g. immune-compromised hosts, sarcoidosis). The relatively more recent interferon-gamma release assay (IGRA) is capable of overcoming some of the drawbacks of the Mantoux test, as it can identify individuals that have been specifically exposed to M. Tuberculosis as opposed to other forms of atypical mycobacteria.

Kumar V, Abbas AK, Fausto N and Mitchell RN. Robbins Basic Pathology, 8th Edition. Saunders Elsevier. 2007, pp. 516-522.

Lawn S and Zumla AI. Tuberculosis. Lancet. 2011;378:57-72.

Pennie RA. Mantoux tests. Performing, interpreting, and acting upon them. Canadian Family Physician. 1995; 41: 1025-29.

32) C: Isoniazid and rifampicin for 6 months, supplemented by pyrazinamide and ethambutol for the first 2 months

RIPE – Rifampicin, Isoniazid, Pyrazinamide and Ethambutol collectively represent the first-line treatment regimen for tuberculosis. Remember *4 for 2, then 2 for 4*; *RIPE* for 2 months, followed by *RI* for 4 months. Thus, rifampicin, isoniazid, pyrazinamide and ethambutol should be used for the first 2 months, followed by only rifampicin and isoniazid for the next 4 months. So, total treatment duration is 6 months. This is the first-line chemotherapy regimen recommended by the International Union Against Tuberculosis and Lung disease, WHO, BTS and NICE guidelines. Note that the emergence of multi-drug resistant (MDR) (resistant to at least rifampicin and isoniazid), and even extensively resistant (XDR) strains of tuberculosis has made the treatment of this condition increasingly challenging.

Prophylaxis of patients infected by TB, but who are completely asymptomatic, is isoniazid for 6 months, or a combination of rifampicin and isoniazid for 3 months.

Lawn S and Zumla AI. Tuberculosis. Lancet. 2011;378:57-72.

Campbell IA and Bah-Sow O. Pulmonary tuberculosis: diagnosis and treatment. British Medical Journal. 2006; 332: 1194-97.

33) D: Ethambutol

All anti-TB drugs can cause liver damage and hepatitis explaining why liver function tests (LFTs) should be routinely monitored.

Ethambutol characteristically causes an optic neuritis and red-green colour blindess. As colour vision is the first to be affected, Ishihara plates are the most sensitive test for ethambutol-mediated optic neuropathy.

Isoniazid increases the risk of peripheral neuropathy and pancreatitis. The use of supplemental pyridoxine (vitamin B6) can help reduce the risk of isoniazid-mediated peripheral neuropathy.

Pyrazinamide is classically associated with gout and joint problems.

Rifampicin characteristically causes a red-orange discolouration of secretions (tears, urine). Rifampicin is an enzyme inducer and can reduce the efficacy of many other drugs.

34) A: It is caused by a mutation in the CFTR gene in chromosome 13

Cystic fibrosis is an autosomal recessive condition caused by mutations, more than 1500 of which have been identified, in the cystic fibrosis transmembrane regulator (CFTR) gene in chromosome 7. Compromised CFTR functions results in reduced secretion of chloride and bicarbonate ions in the respiratory and gastrointestinal tracts, which accounts for abnormally viscid secretions.

Patients are often diagnosed as a result of the national newborn screening programmes. This involves blood spot testing newborns for immunoreactive trypsinogen (IRT). A very high IRT level indicates patients are at risk of CF, but is not 100% specific. If positive, the IRT test is repeated 1-3 weeks later, or alternatively the same original blood sample is tested for the presence of mutations commonly seen in CF. All patients with positive screening results must have the diagnosis of CF confirmed by sweat testing, whereby sweat is induced by pilocarpine iontophoresis – a chloride level of more than 60mmol/l confirms the diagnosis.

Excessively thick pulmonary secretions render patients at increased risk of recurrent lower respiratory tract infections, the end result of which is bronchiectasis, restrictive ventilatory defects (frequently with an obstructive element) and chronic hypoxaemia. Infants with CF are rapidly colonised with Haemophilus influenxa and/ or Staph Aureus. By the age of 3, most infants have serological or culture evidence of Pseudomonas aeruginosa infection. Infection with Burkholderia Cepacia (a complex of at least nine species) later in life can accelerate further deterioration in lung function.

Pulmonary treatment includes the following approaches:

a) *Inhaled hypertonic saline* – helps draw water into the respiratory tract, thereby reducing the viscosity of pulmonary secretions and allowing improved mucociliary clearance of infected debris.

b) *Macrolide antibiotics* – regular prophylactic macrolides (especially azithromycin) has been shown to improve FEV1 and reduce the frequency of pulmonary exacerbations

c) *High dose oral ibuprofen* – mechanism is unclear but has been shown to slow down the rate of deterioration in lung function.

d) *Aggressive treatment of pulmonary exacerbations* – patients with pulmonary exacerbations (demonstrated by deterioration in dyspnoea, cough, sputum production and reduced exercise tolerance) should be admitted and aggressively treated with intravenous antibiotics.

e) *Treatment of co-morbid respiratory conditions* – patients with cystic fibrosis may also suffer from asthma and so should be treated with the relevant inhalers.

f) *Regular daily chest physiotherapy* – in order to aid sputum expectoration and to reduce the frequency of infective exacerbations.

g) *Lung transplantation* – considered as a final therapeutic option in those with end-stage lung disease

Clinical manifestations of cystic fibrosis are legion and are not restricted to pulmonary pathology. These include pancreatic exocrine and endocrine insufficiency, malabsorption, hepatobiliary problems (cholestasis, portal hypertension, liver cirrhosis), bowel obstruction, infertility and more. Consequently, the management of cystic fibrosis as a whole requires a multidisciplinary approach that addresses each and every one of these pathophysiological elements.

O'Sullivan BP and Freedman SD. Cystic Fibrosis. Lancet. 2009; 373: 1891-904

35) E: Ertapenem

This patient has unfortunately developed a Hospital-Acquired Pneumonia (HAP), which is defined as a pneumonia developing more than 48-72 hours after hospital admission. HAP can be split into early and late onset. Early-onset HAP occurs fewer than 5 days following admission to hospital and is more likely to be caused by community-type pathogens susceptible to a greater range of antibiotics. Late-onset HAP, however, occurs after 5 days and tends to be caused by antibiotic-resistant hospital opportunistic pathogens, such as *MRSA* and *Pseudomonas Aeruginosa*.

HAP affects 0.5% to 1.0% of inpatients and is a major cause of morbidity, being estimated to prolong hospital stay by an extra 7-9 days on average. Patients who have had major surgery (e.g. involving a laparotomy) are at particular risk of developing pneumonia because if they don't receive sufficient analgesia, they develop diaphragmatic splinting. Such patients poorly ventilate their lungs, meaning there is a high risk of infection and proliferation of microbial colonies within the airways, leading to pneumonia.

Antibiotics that show high activity against *Pseudomonas Aeruginosa* include piperacillin, tazocin and certain cephaloporins. Pipericillin in combination with the beta-lactamase inhibitor, tazobactam, is Tazocin. Ceftazidime is a third-generation cephalosporin that is highly effective against *Pseudomonas*. Aminoglycosides, such as gentamycin and amikacin act synergistically with other anti-pseudomonal antibiotics; tobramycin, however, is not given to patients with HAP. Tobramycin is often given to patients with cystic fibrosis whom are colonised with *Pseudomonas Aeruginosa*, as a nebuliser in 28-day on and off cycles. Unlike the other carbapenems (meropenem, imipenem and doripenem, which all have good activity against *Pseudomonas*), ertapenem is not active against this pathogen.

Masterton RG, Galloway A, French G et al. Guidelines for the management of hospital-acquired pneumonia in the UK: Report of the Working Party of Hospital-Acquired Pneumonia of the British Society for Antimicrobial Chemotherapy. Journal of Antimicrobial Chemotherapy. 2008;62: 5-34.

British Medical Association and the Royal Pharmaceutical Society of Great Britain. British National Formulary. 62nd ed. UK: BMJ Publishing Group. 2009. Page 346-352

36) B: Extrinsic allergic alveolitis

This patient has farmer's lung, a form of extrinsic allergic alveolitis (also called hypersensitivity pneumonitis), which is both an immune-complex and cell-mediated hypersensitivity reaction (type III and IV, respectively). Patients typically develop symptoms 4-6 hours post-exposure to an antigen they have been sensitised too. Characteristic clinical features include dyspnoea, dry cough, malaise, myalgia, rigors and usually fine bibasal inspiratory crackles with no wheeze. Different forms of extrinsic allergic alveolitis include (but not exhaustive):

a) Farmer's lung – due to exposure to mouldy hay, the major antigen being *Saccharopolyspora rectivirgula* (formerly called *Micropolyspora faeni*)
b) Bird Fancier's lung – due to exposure to avian proteins
c) Malt worker's lung – exposure to *Aspergillus Clavatus* in mouldy malt
d) Mushroom worker's lung – exposure to *Thermophilic Actinomycetes* in mushroom compost
e) Cheese-worker's lung – exposure to cheese mould; *Penicillium casei*
f) Chemical worker's lung – exposure to isocyanates in plastics, paints and resins

Chronic and recurrent exposure to such antigens in particular sensitised individuals can lead to pulmonary fibrosis with a predilection for the upper lobes.

Gulati M. Hypersensitivity Pneumonitis: What's New? American College of Chest Physicians. 2011.

37) C: Churg-Strauss syndrome

Churg-Strauss is one of many eponymous syndromes in medicine and is characterised by a triad of asthma, hyper-eosinophilia and vasculitis, which can potentially affect any organ. This patient has a mononeuritis multiplex (defined as damage to 2 or more peripheral nerves) secondary to vasculitis; inflammation of the vasa nervorum can affect the functioning of the relevantly perfused nerve. In this case, the right superficial peroneal and the left median nerves are affected. Treatment of Churg-Strauss requires a course of high dose steroids (e.g. 40-60mg oral prednisolone once-daily for a month or so to achieve remission, after which the dose is gradually tapered). Young's syndrome is a triad of bronchiectasis, rhino-sinusitis and reduced fertility due to azoospermia in males. Microscopic polyangiitis and wegener's granulomatosis are both vasculitides. Wegener's granulomatosis is a necrotizing granulomatous vasculitis predominantly affecting the upper respiratory tract, lungs and kidneys. Patients may present with destruction of the nasal septum (causing the characteristic 'saddle nose deformity'), sinusitis, epistaxis, pulmonary haemorrhage and rapidly progressive glomerulonephritis.

Microscopic polyangiitis is another type of vasculitis of the small vessels, but like Wegener's, can potentially affect any organ system.

Conron M, Beynon HLC. Churg-Strauss syndrome. Thorax. 2000;55:870-77

38) C: Respiratory alkalosis with metabolic compensation

Whenever interpreting an arterial blood gas, it's always worth bearing in mind the following equilibrium reaction:

$$CO_2 + H_2O \rightleftharpoons H^+ + HCO_3^-$$

The pH of 7.52 makes this an alkalosis (normal pH is 7.35-7.45). The $PaCO_2$ is low. Looking at the above equation, if the $PaCO_2$

drops (for example secondary to hyperventilation), the equilibrium reaction shifts to the left, as there is less carbon dioxide to react with water. This causes the Hydrogen ion concentration to fall, which therefore causes an alkalosis. In order to buffer the pH and bring it back towards the normal value, the equilibrium reaction must shift back towards the right. To do this, the kidneys excrete more bicarbonate ions, lowering the bicarbonate ion concentration, thereby shifting the equilibrium to the right. Thus, the combination of an alkalotic pH, low $PaCO_2$ and low bicarbonate means this is a respiratory alkalosis with metabolic compensation. If the pH was acidic, however, the same bicarbonate and $PaCO_2$ values in this example would be consistent with a metabolic acidosis with respiratory compensation.

Note that it is never possible to overcompensate for a given pH, and that metabolic compensation generally takes significantly longer than respiratory compensation.

Calculating the pH based on the dissociation constant of the equilibrium reaction and the partial pressures/concentrations of the relevant substances in the reaction requires use of the Henderson-Hasselbach equation.

Causes of a respiratory alkalosis include:

a) Psychiatric causes (anxiety, hysteria, stress)
b) CNS causes (stroke, subarachnoid haemorrhage, meningitis)
c) Drug use (doxapram, aspirin, caffeine)
d) High altitude
e) Pregnancy

39) C: Acute respiratory distress syndrome

For a diagnosis of acute lung injury (ALI) to be made, in the appropriate clinical circumstances, the following criteria must be met:

a) Radiological – new bilateral, patchy or diffuse pulmonary infiltrates on a chest X-ray consistent with pulmonary oedema.

b) Pulmonary capillary wedge pressure (an indirect measurement of left atrial pressure) of less than 19mmHg. Higher values suggest pulmonary oedema due to elevated left atrial pressures secondary to left ventricular failure.

c) Refractory hypoxaemia with a PaO2: FiO2 ratio of < 40 kPa

ARDS is a severe form of acute lung injury (ALI) whereby the PaO2: FiO2 ratio is less than 26kPa. Although the patient does have evidence of acute lung injury, ARDS is the more appropriate answer given his severe level of refractory hypoxaemia.

ARDS and ALI have a number of underlying causes including:

a) Pneumonia
b) Aspiration
c) Vasculitis
d) Septicaemia
e) Pancreatitis
f) Trauma
g) Drugs/toxins (e.g. aspirin, paraquat, heroin)
h) Obstetric events (e.g. eclampsia, amniotic fluid embolism)

Ultimately, these all culminate in alveolar inflammation and injury, driving a widespread inflammatory response leading to increased pulmonary capillary permeability and non-cardiogenic pulmonary oedema.

The management of ARDS requires aggressive treatment of the underlying cause and providing general supportive care, often in the ICU setting. Many patients with ARDS will invariably require endotracheal intubation and mechanical ventilation.

Leaver SK and Evans TW. Acute respiratory distress syndrome. British Medical Journal. 2007;335: 389-94

40) E: Chronic obstructive pulmonary disease

This patient has an FEV1: FVC ratio of 50% (i.e. less than 70%, which marks the threshold), indicating an obstructive defect. Of all the conditions listed, only chronic obstructive pulmonary disease (COPD) will produce this spirometry result. The patient's previous occupation and smoking history also places him at significant risk of getting COPD.

COPD is an umbrella term encompassing chronic bronchitis and emphysema. Note that chronic bronchitis is a clinical definition of cough and sputum production on most days for 3 months of 2 consecutive years. Emphysema, however, is defined histopathologically as enlarged air spaces distal to the terminal bronchioles, with alveolar septal destruction.

Cardiology Questions

1) In patients with non-valvular atrial fibrillation, warfarin reduces the rate of ischaemic stroke by approximately how much?

    A. 12-20%
    B. 22-36%
    C. 32-47%
    D. 65-68%
    E. 72-83%

2) A 63-year old gentleman is referred to a cardiologist after his GP incidentally discovers an irregularly irregular pulse during a routine check-up. The patient is otherwise fit and well and is completely asymptomatic. On examination, blood pressure is 128/64 mmHg, pulse is 90/min irregularly irregular, respiratory rate 16/min and temperature 37.2 degrees Celsius.

    What is the single MOST suitable management plan for him?

    A. Commence bisoprolol and anticoagulate with warfarin
    B. Commence bisoprolol and aspirin
    C. Arrange elective electrical DC cardioversion and anticoagulate with warfarin for 2 weeks before and 2 months after procedure
    D. Arrange elective electrical DC cardioversion, and anticoagulate with warfarin for 3 weeks before, and 4 weeks after procedure
    E. Try 'pill-in-the-pocket' approach

3) A 55-year old woman is seen by her GP where she is found to have an irregularly irregular pulse. She is seen 1-week later and is found to have a normal pulse.

    What is the most common presenting symptom for this condition?

    A. Palpitations
    B. Chest pain
    C. Dyspnoea
    D. Syncope
    E. Fatigue

4) A 32-year old female is seen in the medical assessment unit. She has a history of sudden onset pleuritic chest pain and shortness of breath after a flight from Australia. The attending physician requests a 12-lead ECG.

Which of the following is the most common ECG manifestation for this condition?

A. Right bundle branch block
B. Sinus tachycardia
C. Right axis deviation
D. Atrial fibrillation
E. S1Q3T3

5) As part of a first year physiology tutorial a medical student has a 12-lead ECG. He is fit and well with no past medical history.

Where would his cardiac axis be expected to lie?

A. -60 to +90
B. -30 to +90
C. 0 to +90
D. +30 to +90
E. +30 to +120

6) A 92-year old man is clerked by the house officer on-call after presenting with chest pain. He is currently awaiting surgery for colon cancer.

On examination, respiratory rate is 24 breaths per minute, blood pressure is 130/52 mmHg, oxygen saturations 92% on 10L high flow oxygen, pulse is 102 beats per minute (regular) and lung fields are clear to auscultation.

His chest x-ray is unremarkable.

A 12-lead ECG is requested, which reveals evidence of right axis-deviation.

What ECG finding is most consistent with this?

A. Lead I: R wave > S wave, Lead II: R wave = S wave, Lead III: S wave >R wave

B. Lead I: R wave < S wave, Lead II: R wave = S wave, Lead III: R wave > S wave

C. Lead I: S wave = R wave, Lead II: R wave = S wave, Lead III: S wave = R wave

D. Lead I: R wave > S wave, Lead II: R wave = S wave, Lead III: R wave > S wave

E. Lead I: S wave = R wave, Lead II: R wave < S wave, Lead III: S wave = R wave

7) Multiple major randomised-controlled trials have consistently shown that beta-blockers reduce hospitalisation and improve survival, quality of life and NYHA class in patients with stable chronic heart failure.

Which of the following trials has not demonstrated this?

A. USCP
B. MERIT-HF
C. COPERNICUS
D. HOPE
E. CIBIS-II

8) A 71-year old man with chronic heart failure attends a Cardiology Outpatient clinic for a routine follow-up. His current medications include:

Aspirin 75mg OD
Bisoprolol 2.5mg OD
Ramipril 2.5mg OD
Simvastatin 40mg ON
Bendroflumethiazide 2.5mg OD

Which of his medications is least likely to provide a long-term prognostic benefit?

A. Aspirin
B. Bisoprolol
C. Ramipril
D. Simvastatin
E. Bendroflumethiazide

9) A 68-year old male with a 1-hour history of sudden-onset tearing chest pain is seen in Accident and Emergency. He is a known hypertensive, but does not have any other medical problems. On examination, there is an audible early diastolic murmur.

Heart rate:	120/min and regular
Blood pressure:	138/72 mmHg.
12-lead ECG:	ST-segment elevation in leads II, III and aVF.
Troponin T:	1.2 (<0.01ng/ml).

What is the most important diagnostic investigation?

A. Coronary angiography
B. Arterial Blood Gas
C. CT angiography of chest
D. Chest X-ray
E. D-dimer

10) A 50-year old man presents to A&E 7 hours after an episode of central crushing chest pain.

What is the maximum time delay from the onset of chest pain before patients with ST-segment elevation myocardial infarction (STEMI) are no longer considered eligible for primary reperfusion therapy?

A. 2 hours
B. 4 hours
C. 8 hours
D. 12 hours
E. 16 hours

11) A 68-year old female presents to a district general hospital with a 2-hour history of central crushing chest pain, looking pale, sweaty and clammy. She is a heavy smoker with a 40-pack year history and drinks alcohol occasionally. A 12-lead ECG reveals ST-segment elevation of 4mm in leads V1-V4. A decision is made to thrombolyse the patient as she cannot be offered primary PCI in time.

Which ECG features fulfil the criteria for successful reperfusion?

A. A reduction of 1mm of ST-segment elevation after 30 minutes
B. A reduction of 2mm of ST-segment elevation after 30 minutes
C. A reduction of 2mm of ST-segment elevation after 45 minutes
D. A reduction of 1mm of ST-segment elevation after 60 minutes
E. A reduction of 2mm of ST-segment elevation after 60 minutes

12) You are the junior doctor on-call and you see a 76-year old man with an 8-hour history of worsening central chest pain. The pain radiates up his neck into his jaw, and down both arms. There is no history of nausea, clamminess or sweating. He has a 60-pack year history of smoking.

Clinical examination is unremarkable. A 12 lead ECG shows ST-segment depression accompanied by T-wave inversion in leads I, aVL and V6. His renal function is normal.

Which of the following is the MOST appropriate medication that you should prescribe as part of the acute management plan?

A. Aspirin, clopidogrel, glyceryl trinitrate (GTN) spray and morphine PRN
B. Aspirin, clopidogrel, GTN spray and morphine PRN, fondaparinux
C. Aspirin, clopidogrel, GTN spray and morphine PRN, enoxaparin
D. Aspirin, clopidogrel, GTN spray, enoxaparin
E. Aspirin, clopidogrel, GTN spray, fondaparinux

13) After performing a 12-lead ECG on a patient presenting with a 2 hour history of sudden onset epigastric pain, the surgical registrar on-call suspects a case of acute coronary syndrome and immediately calls the medical registrar for help. The medical registrar scrutinises the ECG and sees that the patient may qualify for coronary reperfusion therapy.

Which of the following does not represent an ECG criterion for reperfusion therapy?

A. ST-segment elevation of 2mm in leads V1-V4
B. ST-segment elevation of 1mm in leads V4-V6
C. New-onset Left Bundle Branch Block (LBBB)
D. ST-segment elevation of 1mm in leads II, III and aVF
E. Tall R waves and deep ST-depression in leads V1-V3

14) Your team diagnoses a patient with non-ST segment elevation acute coronary syndrome (NST-ACS).

Which of the following is INCORRECT regarding the management of this condition?

A. Patients should be given a loading dose of 300mg aspirin, followed by 75mg daily
B. Patients with a predicted 6-month mortality < 1.5% do not require clopidogrel
C. Nitrates offer symptomatic relief and carry prognostic benefits
D. Fondaparinux is associated with a lower bleeding risk than therapeutic enoxaparin
E. Glycoprotein IIb/IIIa inhibitors should be considered in patients at intermediate or high risk (predicted 6-month mortality > 3.0%)

15) A 55-year old man is seen in clinic with a high-pitched early diastolic murmur heard best at the left sternal edge in the second intercostal space with the patient in full inspiration.

Which eponymous feature does he have?

A. Duroziez sign
B. Austin-Flint murmur
C. Hill sign
D. Graham-Steell murmur
E. Quincke sign

16) A 68-year old male in the coronary care unit (CCU) develops sudden onset shortness of breath. He was referred to CCU 3 days previously after being thrombolysed for an ST-segment elevation Myocardial Infarction. On examination, the patient looks very unwell, pale, sweaty and severely short of breath.

Auscultation of the chest reveals a pan-systolic murmur radiating to the axilla and bi-basal crepitations.

Heart rate is 130/min and regular
Respiratory rate 26/min
Temperature 37.6 degrees Celsius.

Which of the following complications has occurred?

A. Papillary muscle rupture
B. Ventricular septal wall rupture
C. Cardiac tamponade
D. Ventricular tachycardia
E. Dressler's syndrome

17) A 57-year old lady was recently started on lisinopril following a diagnosis of chronic heart failure secondary to ischaemic heart disease. She is a biology teacher and is concerned about the potential renal toxicity and enquires about the mechanism of this action of ACE inhibitors.

Which of the following regarding the cause of this side effect of ACE inhibitors is correct:

A. Dilatation of renal efferent arterioles
B. Cause an increased susceptibility to renal calculus formation
C. Reduced cardiac output causing pre-renal failure
D. Induce angio-oedema
E. Metabolites cause an acute interstitial nephritis

18) A 53-year old Caucasian male is diagnosed with essential hypertension.

Which of the following is the most appropriate first-line pharmacological treatment?

A. Amlodipine
B. Ramipril
C. Bisoprolol
D. Chlortalidone
E. Furosemide

19) A gentleman with chronic heart failure wants to know which of his medications will not have any effect on his life expectancy. He is breathless at rest and is currently taking atenolol, lisinopril, digoxin, hydralazine, isosorbide mono-nitrate and candesartan. He is being considered for biventricular pacing.

Which of the therapies has no mortality benefit?

A. Hydralazine and nitrates
B. Biventricular pacing
C. Cardiac Glycoside therapy
D. ACE inhibition
E. Beta-Blockade

20) Which of the following is NOT a cardiac cause of digital clubbing?

A. Eisenmenger's syndrome
B. Bacterial endocarditis
C. Atrial myxoma
D. Tetralogy of Fallot
E. Ventricular septal defect

21) A 24-year old man was referred to a cardiologist following a routine medical check-up. He is an army officer and his examination revealed the presence of an incidental systolic murmur on chest examination. After confirming the presence of a pathological murmur, the cardiologist orders an echocardiogram, which demonstrates a significantly enlarged left ventricular wall and inter-ventricular septum.

Which of the following is INCORRECT regarding this patient's condition?

A. Left ventricular outflow tract obstruction is found in approximately 25%   of patients
B. It affects 1 in 500 of the general population
C. Asymmetric hypertrophy occurs in nearly two-thirds of patients
D. The murmur is classically decreased by standing and the valsalva manoeuvre and increased by squatting
E. Giant negative T waves in precordial leads is characteristic of the apical   form of the disease

22) A 72-year old lady presents to her GP with a 5-month history of angina. She is otherwise fit and well and has never smoked. On examination, there is an ejection systolic murmur, with a crescendo-decrescendo quality, radiating to the carotids.

Assuming the absence of any co-morbidities what is the anticipated survival of a patient with this condition without treatment?

A. 1 year
B. 2 years
C. 3 years
D. 5 years
E. 7 years

23) Which of the following patients with aortic stenosis would NOT be eligible for aortic valve replacement surgery?

A. A 73-year old male with a history of syncope and an aortic valve area of 0.5cm²/m² corrected for body surface area (BSA)

B. A 67-year old female with moderate aortic stenosis undergoing coronary artery bypass graft surgery (CABG)

C. A 68-year old asymptomatic, normotensive male with a corrected aortic valve area of 0.5 cm²/m² and left ventricular wall thickness of 17mm

D. A 70-year old female with severe aortic stenosis, asymptomatic at rest but develops angina on exercise testing

E. A 76-year old asymptomatic male with a corrected aortic valve area of 0.8 cm²/m² BSA and a trans-aortic peak velocity progression of 0.1m/s per year

24) You are a medical student in cardiology outpatient's clinic and your consultant asks you to describe the murmur classically heard in mitral stenosis.

Which of the following options is correct?

A. A low pitched rumbling mid-diastolic murmur heard best in the left lateral position with the bell of the stethoscope and breath held in expiration

B. A high pitched rumbling mid-diastolic murmur heard best in the left lateral position with the diaphragm of the stethoscope and breath held in expiration

C. A low pitched rumbling mid-diastolic murmur heard best in the left lateral position with the diaphragm of the stethoscope and breath held in expiration

D. A low pitched rumbling mid-diastolic murmur heard best in the left lateral position with the bell of the stethoscope and breath held in inspiration

E. A high pitched rumbling mid-diastolic murmur heard best in the left lateral position with the bell of the stethoscope and breath held in expiration

25) You perform a cardiovascular examination on a patient and discover that there is a pan-systolic murmur in the lower left sternal border, heard loudest on inspiration.

Which of the following would you expect to find on examination of the patient's Jugular Venous Pressure (JVP)?

A. Cannon a waves
B. Prominent cv waves with a steep y descent
C. Prominent a waves with a steep y descent
D. Pulsatile a waves
E. Steep x descent

26) A 36-year old man presents to Accident and Emergency with a 3-week history of fever, rigors and general malaise. He is well known to the department with complications of intravenous drug abuse.

Clinical examination reveals:
Temperature 39.3 degrees
Heart rate is 120/min
Blood pressure is 122/70 mmHg.,

Cardiovascular examination: early diastolic murmur in the left parasternal line and a left upper quadrant mass is felt on palpation of the abdomen.

Later, a transthoracic echocardiogram demonstrates an aortic root abscess.

Which of the following micro-organisms represents the most likely aetiology for this patient's condition?

A. Streptococcus viridans
B. Coxiella burnetti
C. Coagulase-negative staphylococcus
D. Coagulase-positive staphylococcus
E. Chlamydia psittaci

27) A transthoracic echocardiogram, undertaken in a patient with suspected infective endocarditis, shows evidence of vegetations with prosthetic valve dehiscence. All 3 blood cultures, with the first and last culture taken 1 hour apart, grew Streptococcus Viridans. There is no relevant drug history of note.

Which of the following represents the MOST appropriate first-line antibiotic regimen for this patient?

A. IV benzylpenicillin for 4-6 weeks
B. IV benzylpenicillin and gentamicin for 2-3 weeks
C. IV benzylpenicillin and gentamicin for at least 6 weeks
D. IV vancomycin and gentamicin for at least 6 weeks
E. IV amoxicillin and gentamicin for at least 6 weeks

28) During the morning ward round, your registrar hands over to you a single strip ECG recording taken from a patient, which shows a PR interval of 0.08 seconds.

Which of the following is least likely to represent a cause for this ECG abnormality?

A. Lown-Ganong-Levine (LGL) syndrome
B. Wolff-Parkinson-White (WPW) syndrome
C. Pompe's disease
D. Hypomagnesaemia
E. Fabry's disease

29) You are the on-call house officer clerking a patient who presents with a 1-month history of recurrent palpitations, during which he becomes short of breath and suffers from chest pain and episodes of syncope.

His current medications include Erythromycin, Amitriptyline and Amiodarone. After requesting a 12-lead ECG and performing a quick calculation, you note that the corrected QT-interval is prolonged.

His blood tests show:

Corrected Calcium   2.7 (2.05-2.60mmol/l)
Magnesium   1.3 (1.7 – 2.2mg/dL)

Which of the following does NOT explain this finding?

A. Hypercalcaemia
B. Hypomagnesaemia
C. Erythromycin
D. Amitriptyline
E. Amiodarone

30) Which of the following regarding the antiarrhythmic drug amiodarone is INCORRECT?

A. The elimination half-life of oral amiodarone therapy is 50-60 days
B. Amiodarone has class I, II, III and IV antiarrhythmic activity
C. Amiodarone increases serum digoxin levels and potentiates the anticoagulant effects of warfarin
D. In the Sudden Cardiac Death in Heart Failure Trial (SCD-HeFT) amiodarone was superior to placebo in improving survival among heart failure patients
E. Between 1-2% of patients on long-term amiodarone develop a grey-bluish skin discoloration

31) A 32-year old female presents to A and E with a 1-hour history of palpitations. Past medical history includes severe asthma requiring multiple hospitalisations. On examination, the patient looks anxious.

Breath sounds are normal bilaterally with good air entry. Blood pressure is 126/84 mmHg.

A 12-lead ECG is performed, which demonstrates a regular narrow-complex tachycardia with a rate of 190/min.

Carotid massage and valsalva manoeuvres fail to terminate the arrhythmia.

Which of the following represents the next most appropriate form of management?

A. Synchronised DC cardioversion
B. Adenosine 6mg bolus, followed by 12mg if unsuccessful
C. 2.5mg intravenous atenolol at a rate of 1mg/minute
D. 2.5-5mg verapamil given intravenously over 2 minutes
E. Amiodarone 300mg intravenously over 20-60 minutes followed by 900mg over 24 hours

32) Which of the following statements regarding the coronary arteries and venous drainage of the heart is INCORRECT?

A. The left coronary artery originates from the left posterior aortic sinus
B. The posterior descending artery represents a branch of the right coronary artery in up to 60% of individuals
C. The right coronary artery supplies the atrioventricular node in approximately 90% of individuals
D. The coronary sinus drains venous blood into the right atrium
E. Thebesian veins are responsible for 20-30% of all venous drainage

33) A 43-year old gentleman on lipid lowering therapy for ischaemic heart disease presents with a 2-day history of progressively worsening muscular pain. His drug history (past and present) includes:

Simvastatin, Clarithromycin, Amiodarone, Ciclosporin, Itraconazole and Furosemide.

Which of the following drug pairs is LEAST likely to have precipitated this patient's symptoms?

A. Simvastatin and clarithromycin
B. Simvastatin and amiodarone
C. Simvastatin and ciclosporin
D. Simvastatin and itraconazole
E. Simvastatin and furosemide

34) A 70-year old woman is brought to A and E by her daughter who is concerned that her mother has become increasingly confused lately. The patient has a history of heart failure and is on Furosemide 80mg,

Bendroflumethiazide 2.5mg, Ramipril 2.5mg, Bisoprolol 7.5mg and Digoxin 125 micrograms, all taken orally once a day.

Her daughter also claims that her mother has suffered from nausea, vomiting and had complained of seeing yellow-green halos around objects.

On examination:

Heart rate	48/min and regular
Blood pressure	110/76 mmHg
Respiratory rate	16/min
Oxygen saturation	98% on air
Temperature	37.2 degrees Celcius

Which of the following is the most likely diagnosis?

A. Bisoprolol toxicity due to hypokalaemia
B. Digoxin toxicity due to hyponatraemia
C. Digoxin toxicity due to hypokalaemia
D. Bisoprolol toxicity due to hypocalcaemia
E. Digoxin toxicity due to hyperkalaemia

35) A new biomarker is being assessed for its use as a predictor for the development of chronic heart failure. In a trial that included 220 patients at risk of heart failure, 140 actually developed the condition. Of those that developed heart failure, 40 of them tested negative for the biomarker.

What is the sensitivity of this test?

A. 71%
B. 76%
C. 79%
D. 82%
E. 85%

36) A particular type of pacemaker functions by delivering regular electrical stimuli to the ventricles, inducing ventricular contraction. If the ventricles contract spontaneously, then the pacemaker output is inhibited during that time period.

Which of the following three-letter combination describes the aforementioned pacemaker?

A. VVI
B. VIV
C. IVV
D. DDD
E. DDI

Cardiology Answers

1) **D: 65-68%**

Systematic reviews of randomised controlled trials have shown that in patients with non-valvular atrial fibrillation (AF):

a) Aspirin reduces the risk of stroke by 22-36% compared with placebo
b) Warfarin reduces the risk of stroke by 65-68% compared with placebo and 32-47% compared with aspirin.

The use of risk stratification scoring systems (CHADS2 and CHA2DS2-VASC) can inform clinicians of those groups of patients whom are most likely to benefit from anticoagulation therapy.

Congestive heart failure – 1 point
Hypertension – 1 point
Age > 75 years – 1 point
Diabetes mellitus – 1 point
(History of) **S**troke or TIA – 2 points

A score of 2 or more: anticoagulation with warfarin is recommended
A score of 1: aspirin or warfarin
A score of 0: aspirin or no anticoagulation considered

The more recent CHA2DS2-VASC scoring system incorporates more variables known to contribute to increased stroke risk in AF, namely vascular disease and female sex, and places increased weight on age (age>75 years: 2 points, age 65-74 years: 1 point).

Olesen JB, Lip GYH, Hansen ML, Hansen PR, Tolstrup JS, Lindhardsen J et al. Validation of risk stratification schemes for predicting stroke and thromboembolism in patients with atrial fibrillation: nationwide cohort study. British Medical Journal. 2011;342:d124

Lafuente-Lafuente C, Mahe I and Extramiana F. Management of atrial fibrillation. British Medical Journal. 2009;339: 40-45

2) D: Arrange elective electrical cardioversion, and anticoagulate with warfarin for 3 weeks before, and 4 weeks after procedure

The management of atrial fibrillation (AF) can be targeted towards controlling heart rate and preventing the occurrence of fast AF ('rate control') or towards the restoration of sinus rhythm ('rhythm control').

Atrial fibrillation (AF) can be classified into:

a) *Paroxysmal* – lasts < 7 days duration (usually <48 hours), which terminates spontaneously

b) *Persistent* – lasts > 7 days, requiring cardioversion (chemical or electrical) to restore sinus rhythm as it rarely terminates spontaneously

c) *Permanent* – restoration of sinus rhythm is no longer considered feasible due to previous multiple unsuccessful attempts at cardioversion

Rhythm control is the preferred option in paroxysmal AF, whereas rate control is preferred in permanent AF. Persistent AF may merit either rate or rhythm control. However, the precise management plan must be tailored to each individual patient, taking into consideration patient preference, co-morbidities, number of previous failed attempts at cardioversion and any existing contraindications to rate or rhythm control strategies.

Given the patient's condition in this clinical scenario, that he is generally fit and well with no co-morbidities and no previous failures at cardioversion, rhythm control would be the desired therapeutic strategy.

According to NICE guidelines, if AF onset is < 48 hours ago, the patient can be cardioverted without delay under heparin cover, with no further anticoagulation necessary. However, if the onset is > 48 hours ago or if the time of onset is unclear, elective electrical cardioversion can be arranged, with warfarin anticoagulation required for 3 weeks before and 4 weeks after the procedure. The reason for such anticoagulation cover is that cardioversion runs the risk of dislodging an atrial thrombus into the systemic circulation; this thrombus is more likely to be present the longer a patient remains in AF. If cardioversion cannot be delayed, then it should be performed promptly under heparin cover, providing a trans-oesophageal echocardiogram has excluded an atrial thrombus.

National Institute for Health and Clinical Excellence (2006). Atrial Fibrillation: National clinical guideline for management in primary and secondary care. CG36. London: National Institute for Health and Clinical Excellence.

3) **A: Palpitations**

National Institute for Health and Clinical Excellence (2006). Atrial Fibrillation: National clinical guideline for management in primary and secondary care. CG36. London: National Institute for Health and Clinical Excellence.

4) **B: Sinus tachycardia**

See respiratory chapter for a description of pulmonary embolism.

5) **B: -30 to +90.**

6) **B: Lead I: R wave < S wave, Lead II: R wave = S wave, Lead III: R wave > S wave**

The type of cardiac axis deviation can be identified by scrutinizing the limb leads, whilst bearing in mind their recording orientations and the fact that the normal cardiac axis range is -30 to +90 degrees. Lead I is orientated at 0 degrees, lead II is orientated at +60 degrees and lead III is orientated at +120 degrees.

If the R wave equals the S wave, then it means that the direction of ventricular depolarisation is oriented at right angles to the recording lead. If the magnitude of the R wave exceeds the S wave, then it means the wave of depolarisation is directed, on average, towards the recording lead (less than 90 degrees). If the magnitude of the R wave is smaller than the S wave, then the wave of ventricular depolarisation is propagating away from the recording lead on average (more than 90 degrees).

Thus, in right axis deviation, the wave of ventricular depolarisation should be from +90 degrees to +180 degrees (or as far as (patho) physiologically possible). This means that this wave is more than 90 degrees away from lead I (hence R wave < S wave) and towards the direction of lead III (hence R wave > S wave). In this specific answer option, the R wave = S wave in lead II, meaning that the wave of ventricular depolarisation is oriented at right angles to lead II, thereby suggesting the specific cardiac axis is, in actual fact, +150 degrees.

7) **D: HOPE**

USCP = United States Carvedilol Programme
MERIT-HF = Metoprolol CR/XL Randomised Intervention Trial in Heart Failure trial
COPERNICUS = Carvedilol Prospective Randomized Cumulative Survival trial
CIBIS-II = Cardiac Insufficiency Bisoprolol Study II

The HOPE (Heart Outcomes Prevention Evaluation) study showed that the ACE-inhibitor ramipril reduces all-cause mortality, cardiovascular events and nephropathy in patients with diabetes.

8) **E: Bendroflumethiazide**

9) **C: CT angiography of chest**

Although this patient suffered from an inferior myocardial infarction, thrombolysis would probably have killed him, as this was secondary to an acute aortic dissection. In this scenario, the dissection was type A (see below), which propagated proximally, affecting the aortic valve (explaining the early diastolic murmur of aortic regurgitation) and the coronary arteries (in this case, right coronary dissection explains the inferior ST elevation myocardial infarction).

Key features that should raise suspicion of an acute aortic dissection are:

1) Classical history of a 'tearing' or 'ripping' chest pain, which may radiate to the neck or back.
2) Examination features – new aortic regurgitation, pulse delays and/or blood pressure discrepancies between opposite limbs.
3) Symptoms/signs of end-organ malperfusion – acute limb/visceral/cerebral/myocardial ischaemia or infarction. Look for relevant signs, e.g. neurological in case dissection has spread to carotids.

European Society of Cardiology guidelines recommend that in patients with suspected acute aortic dissection, the first-line investigation is a multidetector CT angiography of the chest.

Management depends mainly on the location and extent of the dissection. Aortic dissections can be classified as type A or B, according to the Stanford classification. Type A dissections involve the ascending aorta (alone or with descending aortic co-involvement), whereas type B dissections are restricted to the descending aorta, defined as distal to the origin of the left subclavian artery. Type A dissections are managed surgically, whereas uncomplicated type B dissections (i.e. pain or hypertension responsive to medical treatment and with no acute limb/visceral ischaemia) are managed conservatively through careful regulation of blood pressure.

Left untreated, acute aortic dissection carries an exceptionally high mortality. In the case of type A dissections, mortality rate increases by 1-2% per hour in the first day and approaches 90% at 30 days, explaining why prompt diagnosis and management is imperative for this rare, but very serious condition.

Ranasinghe AM, Strong D, Boland B and Bonser RS. Acute aortic dissection. British Medical Journal. 2011;343:d4487

Thrumurthy SG, Karthikesalingam A, Patterson BO, Holt PJE and Thompson MM. The diagnosis and management of aortic dissection. British Medical Journal. 2011;344:d8290

10) D: 12 hours

Reperfusion therapy for STEMI encompasses fibrinolytic therapy (thrombolysis) and primary percutaneous coronary intervention (primary PCI) with the goal of re-establishing coronary perfusion and salvaging viable myocardium at the brink of infarction.

Although the superiority of primary PCI over fibrinolytic therapy is well established, the benefits of both forms of reperfusion therapies fall rapidly with time. Primary PCI is preferred within 90-120 minutes of first medical contact, but as this can be logistically challenging, fibrinolytic therapy is preferred in those patients presenting within 3 hours of chest pain onset and whom cannot be offered primary PCI within the desired time frame. Beyond 12 hours of the onset of chest pain, little benefit from either form of reperfusion therapy is seen.

Keeley EC and Hillis DL. Primary PCI for Myocardial Infarction with ST-Segment Elevation. The New England Journal of Medicine. 2007;356;1:47-54

Keeley EC, Boura JA, Grines CL. Primary angioplasty versus intravenous thrombolytic therapy for acute myocardial infarction: a quantitative review of 23 randomised trials. Lancet 2003; 361: 13e20.

11) E: A reduction of 2mm of ST-segment elevation after 60 minutes

The patient with STEMI who is thrombolysed is considered to be successfully reperfused if there is a resolution of at least 50% of the initial ST-segment elevation on a follow-up ECG performed 60-90 minutes after thrombolysis. More than 70% resolution would suggest complete reperfusion. Failure to reperfuse following thrombolysis may necessitate 'rescue' PCI, providing patients have presented within 6 hours of symptom onset of STEMI.

Shelton RJ and Blackman DJ. Management of ST-elevation myocardial infarction. Medicine. 2010; 38(8): 431-437

Scottish Intercollegiate Guidelines Network (2007). Acute Coronary Syndromes. Guideline No. 93.

12) B: Aspirin, clopidogrel, GTN spray and morphine PRN, fondaparinux

This patient has a non-ST-segment elevation acute coronary syndrome (NST-ACS), with involvement of the lateral myocardium. Until the results of a cardiac biomarker test (e.g. troponin T or I performed 12 hours after symptom onset) is known, it is not possible to discern whether the cause of this patient's problem is unstable angina or an NSTEMI. Either way, the acute management plan for both conditions is the same. As well as standard resuscitative measures (e.g. oxygen), patients with NST-ACS require:

1) *Anti-platelet therapy*– a 300mg loading dose of **aspirin** and **clopidogrel** is given initially. From the following day, 75mg daily aspirin should continue indefinitely and, unless the patient is at low risk of further ischaemic events, 75mg clopidogrel should also be given daily, but for a limited time period (usually 12 months, but this depends on the level of risk and on stent placement).

2) *Anti-ischaemic therapy* – **nitrates**, which preferentially cause venodilation to reduce myocardial preload and oxygen demand, and coronary vasodilation to improve myocardial oxygen supply. Unless the patient is haemodynamically unstable, **beta-blockers** should also be commenced immediately to prevent further ischaemia by virtue of their negative chronotropic and inotropic properties.

3) *Anticoagulants* – Fondaparinux (an anti-Xa pentasaccharide) is preferable to low molecular weight heparins as they are associated with a lower risk of major bleeding and mortality (results of the OASIS-5 trial).

Patients with evidence of recurrent ischaemia will also require prompt coronary angiography (within 24-96 hours), with revascularisation (PCI or coronary artery bypass grafting) if needed, providing they are at intermediate to high risk of further cardiovascular events. The patient's risk can be quantified as 6-month mortality rate predictions using recognised scoring systems such as the GRACE risk model. If the patient is considered to be at low risk of further coronary events, then a cardiac stress test, such as an exercise tolerance test, should be arranged. Coronary angiography (with or without revascularisation) would then be recommended if inducible myocardial ischaemia occurs during stress testing. Given the clear ischaemic ECG changes in this patient along with the classical history of cardiac chest pain, it would be appropriate to proceed straight to coronary angiography. Educating the patient, encouraging smoking cessation and starting statins and ACE inhibitors should also form part of a secondary prevention management strategy.

Henderson RA. Ischaemic heart disease: management of non-ST-elevation acute coronary syndrome. Medicine. 2010;38:424-430

Peters RJG, Mehta S and Yusuf S. Acute coronary syndromes without ST segment elevation. British Medical Journal. 2007;334: 1265-1269

National Institute for Health and Clinical Excellence (2010). Unstable angina and NSTEMI. CG94. London: National Institute for Health and Clinical Excellence.

13) *B:* ST-segment elevation of 1mm in leads V4-V6

The following are ECG criteria for reperfusion therapy (thrombolysis or primary PCI):

a) ST-segment elevation of at least 2mm in 2 or more contiguous chest leads
b) ST-segment elevation of at least 1mm in 2 or more contiguous limb leads
c) New onset LBBB
d) ECG features raising the possibility of posterior infarction (deep ST depression and tall R waves in the anterior chest leads) – in practice this will necessitate attaching posterior chest leads on the patient for verification.

This case scenario also illustrates the importance of performing a 12-lead ECG on a patient presenting with acute epigastric pain – a case designated an acute abdomen and referred to the surgeons may in fact be an acute coronary syndrome requiring the medics!

14) C: Nitrates offer symptomatic relief and carry prognostic benefits

Both unstable angina and non-ST elevation myocardial infarction (NSTEMI) are grouped under the rubric non-ST elevation acute coronary syndromes (NST-ACS).

Nitrates solely offer symptomatic relief and do not confer any reduction in mortality or improvements in prognosis in acute coronary syndromes.

The OASIS-5 trial showed that fondaparinux (2.5mg s.c. once daily) and enoxaparin (1mg/kg s.c. twice daily) were associated with similar rates of ischaemic events at 9 days, but fondaparinux halved the risk of major bleeding.

Certain scoring systems such as GRACE (Global Registry of Acute Coronary Events) can be used to compute 6-month mortality rates in patients with NST-ACS. These figures can then be used to guide treatment and target more intensive therapies to those patient groups at greater risk of further ischaemic events.

National Institute for Health and Clinical Excellence (2010). Unstable angina and NSTEMI. CG94. London: National Institute for Health and Clinical Excellence.

Henderson RA. Ischaemic heart disease: management of non-ST-elevation acute coronary syndrome. Medicine. 2010;38:424-430

15) D: Graham-Steell murmur

This is associated with pulmonary regurgitation. Although of limited practical value, at least for aortic/pulmonary regurgitation, eponymous signs are an examiner's favourite!

Graham-Steell murmur describes the pulmonary regurgitation that can occur secondary to pulmonary arterial hypertension. The remaining epnonyms are signs of aortic regurgitation:

a)   Duroziez sign – systolic and diastolic to-and-fro femoral murmurs auscultated when the femoral artery is compressed.
b)   Austin-Flint murmur – the mid-to-late diastolic murmur occurring in aortic regurgitation. Although several theories have been posited, one theory suggests that it occurs as a result of the aortic regurgitant jet impinging on the mitral valve leaflets during diastole, resulting in a functional mitral stenosis. The murmur therefore mimics that of mitral stenosis and is heard best using the bell of the stethoscope with the patient lying in the left lateral position. By definition, an Austin-Flint murmur cannot occur in patients with mitral stenosis.
c)   Hill sign – describes the increased manually measured blood pressure in the lower limbs compared with the upper limbs in some patients with aortic regurgitation.
d)   Quincke's sign – exaggerated capillary pulsations of the nail beds.

Another eponym worth learning is Corrigan's sign, which describes the abrupt distension and collapse of the carotid pulse in aortic regurgitation.

Babu AN, Kymes SM and Fryer SMC. Eponyms and the Diagnosis of Aortic Regurgitation: What Says the Evidence? Annals of Internal Medicine. 2003;138:736-42.

16) A: Papillary muscle rupture

The patient has acute left ventricular failure secondary to acute mitral regurgitation, which had arisen due to papillary muscle rupture rendering the mitral valves incompetent. Ventricular septal rupture can also cause new-onset pan-systolic murmur post-myocardial infarction, but the murmur would not radiate to the axilla.

Cardiac tamponade can occur after a myocardial infarction if the ventricular free wall ruptures causing a haemopericardium.

Ischaemic heart disease and previous myocardial infarctions collectively represent the most common cause of ventricular tachycardia, but heart rates of over 150/min would be expected.

Dressler's syndrome is a rare autoimmune phenomenon, secondary to myocardial injury (e.g. myocardial infarction, cardiac surgery etc), and manifests itself as pleuritis, pericarditis and fever several weeks to months after the primary insult. The chief presenting complaint would therefore be pleuritic or pericarditic chest pain (sharp, localised, worse on inspiration and in pericarditis, worse on lying down and relieved by sitting forward), often accompanied by malaise and reduced appetite, with or without shortness of breath due to pleural effusion.

Horenstein SM and Berger S. Postpericardiotomy Syndrome. eMedicine. 2012.

17) A: Dilatation of renal efferent arterioles

Angiotensin II constricts renal efferent arterioles in preference to afferent arterioles, which maintains the pressure gradient required for driving glomerular filtration. ACE inhibitors inhibit the Angiotensin Converting Enzyme (ACE), thereby reducing angiotensin II levels. This leads to reduced renal efferent arteriolar constriction (i.e. a relative dilation), causing GFR to drop. This explains why ACE inhibitors often cause a rise in creatinine shortly after starting the drug, and why doses should be increased gradually (not less than 2 weekly intervals) with regular monitoring of renal function (before and after dose changes). A rise in creatinine of less than 50% of baseline is acceptable. If the creatinine rise is 50-100% of baseline, then the dose must be halved, whereas if it is more than 100%, then the ACE inhibitor should be stopped altogether.

The most common side effect of ACE inhibitors is dry cough, which is believed to be due to reduced breakdown of bradykinin. As ACE inhibitors are anti-hypertensives, hypotension is not surprisingly another adverse drug reaction. First dose hypotension effects mean that ACE inhibitors should be taken at night during the start of treatment. Another problem is hyperkalaemia since ACE inhibitors lower aldosterone levels, the secretion of which is normally stimulated by angiotensin II. In the context of heart failure, hyperkalaemia may be exacerbated by co-existing renal dysfunction and the possible co-prescription of potassium-sparing diuretics, such as amiloride and spironolactone. Thus, electrolytes should routinely be measured in patients on ACE inhibitor therapy.

Walsh K. Heart failure: an update on management. BMJ learning

Davies MK, Gibbs CR and Lip GY. ABC of heart failure. Management: diuretics, ACE inhibitors, and nitrates. British Medical Journal. 2000;320:428-31.

McMurray J, Cohen-Solal A, Dietz R, Eichhorn E, Erhardt L, Hobbs FD et al. Practical recommendations for the use of ACE inhibitors, beta-blockers, aldosterone antagonists and angiotensin receptor blockers in heart failure: putting guidelines into practice. European Journal of Heart Failure. 2005;7:710-21.

18) B: Ramipril

According to NICE guidelines, patients over the age of 55 years should receive calcium channel blockers, whilst patients under 55 should receive ACE inhibitors as first-line treatment. Black people of African or Caribbean origin of any age, however, should receive calcium channel blockers first line. Should these measures fail to resolve hypertension, a combination of ACE inhibitors and calcium channel blockers should be used as second-line treatment, followed by the addition of a diuretic if blood pressure still remains high.

It should be noted that there has been much controversy surrounding the most recent NICE guidelines for the management of hypertension, with critics arguing that:

1) The now recommended use of ambulatory and home blood pressure monitoring in preference to clinic measurements for diagnosing hypertension lacks sufficient evidence base
2) The new threshold for diagnosing and monitoring hypertension is too high
3) The relegation of diuretics from first to third-line management is not sound, as their evidence of effectiveness is among the best for any drug treatment
4) And the new recommendation of chlortalidone and indapamide in preference to bendroflumethiazide and hydrochlorothiazide diuretics also lacks sufficient evidence.

National Institute for Health and Clinical Excellence (2006). Hypertension. CG34. London: National Institute for Health and Clinical Excellence.

National Institute for Health and Clinical Excellence (2011). Hypertension. CG127. London: National Institute for Health and Clinical Excellence.

Brown MJ, Cruickshank JK and MacDonald TM. Navigating the shoals in hypertension: discovery and guidance. British Medical Journal. 2012;344:d8218

McManus RJ, Caulfield M and Williams B. NICE hypertension guideline 2011: evidence based evolution. British Medical Journal. 2012;344:e181

19) C: Cardiac Glycoside therapy

The DIG (Digitalis Investigation Group) study showed that digoxin reduced hospital admission rates in chronic heart failure, but conferred no significant reduction in overall mortality. ACE inhibitors and beta-blockers, which represent the pharmacological cornerstone of chronic heart failure management, have been consistently proven to reduce patient morbidity and mortality. Diuretics are used for symptomatic management, but have no prognostic benefit.

Biventricular pacing (also known as Cardiac Resynchronisation Therapy (CRT)) is indicated for patients who are in sinus rhythm and have class III or ambulatory class IV heart failure with evidence of poor ejection fraction (<35%) despite optimal medical treatment. The aim of CRT is to rectify the loss of ventricular synchrony that compromises pump function in heart failure, and has been shown by the CARE HF study to reduce all-cause mortality by 36%, when used with drug therapy, compared with medical treatment alone.

A significant cause of death in heart failure is ventricular arrhythmias. Certain groups of heart failure patients may qualify for Implantable Cardioverter Defibrillators (ICD), which are designed to recognise and terminate, by appropriately shocking, life-threatening ventricular arrhythmias. Studies have shown that in conjunction with optimal medical therapy, ICDs can reduce mortality by 23-31%. Interestingly, the COMPANION trial has shown the incremental mortality benefits of combining CRT with ICD in certain selected groups of patients with chronic heart failure.

Bristow MR, Feldman AM, Saxon LA. Heart failure management using implantable devices for ventricular resynchronization: Comparison of Medical Therapy, Pacing, and Defibrillation in Chronic Heart Failure (COMPANION) trial. J Card Fail 2000;
6: *276–85.*

Bristow MR, Saxon LA, Boehmer J, et al. Cardiac-resynchronization therapy with or without an implantable defibrillator in advanced chronic heart failure. N Engl J Med 2004; **350:** *2140–50.*

Cleland JGF, Daubert J-C, Erdmann E, et al. The effect of cardiac resynchronization on morbidity and mortality in heart failure. New England Journal of Medicine 2005; **352:** *1539–49.*

Digitalis Investigation Group. The effect of digoxin on mortality and morbidity in patients with heart failure. New England Journal of Medicine 1997; **336:** *525–33.*

Krum H and Abraham WT. Heart failure. The Lancet. 2009;373:941-955

20) E: Ventricular septal defect

Cardiac causes of clubbing:
- **A**trial myxoma
- **B**acterial endocarditis
- **C**yanotic heart disease

Ventricular septal defect *per se* is not a cause of clubbing. Only when the initial left-right shunt converts to a right-left shunt (i.e. Eisenmenger's syndrome), so that a cyanotic heart disease results, will digital clubbing develop.

21) D: The murmur is classically decreased by standing and the valsalva manoeuvre and increased by squatting

Hypertrophic cardiomyopathy (HCM) is commonly picked up incidentally, although patients may present with a history of dyspnoea, chest pain or syncope. HCM is also a well-recognised cause of sudden cardiac death, secondary to life-threatening ventricular arrhythmias. Patients must therefore be assessed for an implantable cardioverter-defibrillator based on their risk for sudden death.

Clinical findings characteristic of HCM, and not uncommonly asked in exams, include a jerky carotid pulse, double apical impulse, fourth heart sound and a late ejection systolic murmur, which is increased by manoeuvres that reduce preload or afterload, like standing and the valsalva manoeuvre and decreased by squatting (since the latter increases both preload and afterload).

Soor GS, Luk A, Ahn E, Abraham JR, Woo A, Ralph-Edwards A and Butany J. Hypertrophic cardiomyopathy: current understanding and treatment objectives. Journal of Clinical Pathology. 2009;62:226-235

Elliott P and McKenna WJ. Hypertrophic cardiomyopathy. Lancet. 2004;363:1881-91.

22) D: 5 years

The onset of angina, syncope or heart failure, which indicates the presence of severe symptomatic aortic stenosis, carries a predicted average survival of 5, 3 and 2 years, respectively.

Although aortic stenosis frequently co-exists with coronary artery disease, patients with aortic stenosis can still suffer from angina in the presence of normal coronary arteries. This is due to a combination of the increased myocardial oxygen demand of the hypertrophied pressure-overloaded left ventricle, and a compromised coronary supply (due to high diastolic filling pressures compressing endocardium and reduced capillary density).

Carabello BA and Paulus WJ. Aortic stenosis. Lancet. 2009;373:956-66

23) E: A 76 year old asymptomatic male with a corrected aortic valve area of 0.8 cm²/m² BSA and a transaortic peak velocity progression of 0.1m/s per year

The presence of severe aortic stenosis (absolute aortic valve orifice area of <1cm² or < 0.6cm²/m² BSA or aortic gradient of > 40mmHg) in conjunction with symptoms (angina/syncope/heart failure) or certain other criteria (e.g. symptoms provoked on exercise testing, LV ejection fraction <50%, peak trans-aortic velocity progression > 0.3 m/s per year etc) requires surgical intervention in the form of aortic valve replacement. Valve replacement can also be considered in patients with moderate stenosis whom are already undergoing CABG (see ESC guidelines for further indications).

More recent technological developments have permitted the consideration of operating on higher risk patients, such as those with multiple severe co-morbidities, via percutaneous methods (transcatheter aortic valve replacement).

Vahanian A, Baumgartner H, Bax J, Butchart E, Dion R, Fillipatos G et al. Guidelines on the management of valvular heart disease: the Task Force on the Management of Valvular Heart Disease of the European Society of Cardiology. European Heart Journal. 2007;28:230–68.

Holmes DR, Mack MJ, Kaul S, Agnihotri A, Alexander KP, Bailey SR et al. 2012 ACCF/AATS/SCAI/STS Expert Consensus Document on Transcatheter Aortic Valve Replacement. Journal of the American College of Cardiology. 2012;59:1200-54.

24) A: A low pitched rumbling mid-diastolic murmur heard best in the left lateral position with the bell of the stethoscope and breath held in expiration

Knowledge of the murmurs associated with different valvular heart lesions are commonly asked during finals.

Aortic stenosis characteristically produces an ejection mid-systolic murmur, with a crescendo-decrescendo quality, radiating to the carotids.

Aortic regurgitation (AR) produces an early diastolic murmur with a decrescendo quality, loudest at the left sternal edge. An ejection systolic murmur may also be heard in AR as the regurgitant jet adds to the subsequent left ventricular end-diastolic volume, increasing ventricular stretch and boosting ejection flow, resulting in a flow murmur during the next systolic phase (the Frank-Starling principle). Furthermore, the regurgitant blood flow in early diastole can impinge on the mitral valve leaflets, producing a functional mitral stenosis, which may cause a mid-diastolic murmur in severe AR (Austin-Flint murmur).

Mitral regurgitation classically produces a pan-systolic murmur with a 'blowing' quality, radiating to the axilla.

Note that all of the aforementioned murmurs (with the exception of mitral stenosis) are high-pitched, and therefore heard best with the diaphragm of the stethoscope. Additionally, all murmurs produced by left-sided valvular heart lesions are accentuated with the breath held in expiration. The reason for this is that in inspiration, the negative intra-thoracic pressure, combined with a raised intra-abdominal pressure (due to downward diaphragmatic movement), creates a pressure gradient that enhances venous return to the right side of the heart, at the expense of the left side.

Concurrently, pulmonary venous return to the left side of the heart is reduced (partly because of blood pooling in the lungs), which reduces the magnitude of left-sided trans-valvular blood flow, thereby decreasing left sided murmurs. Expiration has the opposite effect.

Kumar P and Clark M. Kumar and Clark's Clinical Medicine, Seventh Edition. 2009.

Kirby B and MacLeod K. Clinical examination of the heart. Medicine. 2006;34:123-128.

25) B: Prominent cv waves with a steep y descent

For the purposes of performing a cardiovascular examination during the OSCEs, it would suffice to simply identify whether the JVP is elevated or not. Questions concerning abnormalities of specific components of the JVP waveform are more likely to come up in the written examinations.

As the internal jugular vein lies in continuity with the right atrium, with the absence of intervening valves, the Jugular Venous Pressure (JVP) can be used as an indirect marker of right atrial pressure. Below is an explanation of the different waveform components of the JVP wave written in the order they arise:

a wave – corresponds to atrial contraction
c wave – approximates to the period of isovolumetric contraction, where the closed tricuspid valve 'bulges' into the right atrium as the right intraventricular pressure rises, before the pulmonary valves have opened
x decent – atrial volume increases due to a combination of atrial relaxation and the tricuspid valve 'rebounding' back towards the right ventricular cavity as blood is ejected into the pulmonary circulation during ventricular systole.
v wave – right atrium fills with blood whilst the tricuspid valve remains closed
y decent – right atrium empties as the tricuspid valve opens (not as steep as the x decent in normal conditions).

The patient in this scenario has tricuspid regurgitation (recall that right-sided heart murmurs are louder on inspiration), producing large cv waves. Cannon a waves can occur in atrioventricular dissociation (e.g. complete heart block) because when the atrial contractions coincide with the ventricular contractions, the right atrium slams blood into a closed tricuspid valve sporadically producing larger cannon-like a waves. Steep y descents can be seen in constrictive pericarditis as well as tricuspid regurgitation.

Senguttuvan NB and Karthikeyan G. Jugular Venous C-V Wave in Severe Tricuspid Regurgitation. The New England Journal of Medicine. 2012;366:e5

Ashley EA, Niebauer J. Cardiology Explained. London: Remedica; 2004. Cardiovascular examination

26) D: Coagulase-positive staphylococcus

Despite modern advances in non-invasive imaging, diagnostic protocols and therapeutic strategies, infective endocarditis still carries a high annual mortality, approaching 40%. The most common clinical presentation is **fever** (up to 90% of patients), often arising in association **with rigors, anorexia and weight loss**. Other symptoms and signs include:

1) **Hands** - digital clubbing, splinter haemorrhages, Osler's nodes (tender nodules on finger pulps), Janeway lesions (non-tender palmar/plantar purpura)
2) **Retina** – Roth spots
3) **Heart** – valvular incompetence
4) **Neurological deficits** – stroke/TIA, due to vascular phenomena spanning major arterial emboli, mycotic aneurysms and intracranial haemorrhages
5) **Kidneys** – Glomerulonephritis producing micro- or macroscopic haematuria
6) **Splenomegaly**
7) **Blood** – positive blood cultures, rheumatoid factor

Intravenous (IV) drug users are at increased risk of infective endocarditis compared with the general population (incidence of 1-5% per year vs 0.0017 -0.0062% per year, respectively). Among IV drug users, right-sided and left-sided valvular lesions occur with equal frequency. The finding that right sided lesions are more commonly seen in IV drug users, however, may be explained by the fact that infective endocarditis is more common within this high-risk group.

Staphylococcus aureus (a coagulase-positive staphylococcus) is the most common culprit among IV drug users, whilst Streptococcus viridans is most common in the general population.

Diagnosis of endocarditis can be made using the Modified Duke Criteria (see references below for more information). Blood cultures represent the single most important investigation in endocarditis (followed by transthoracic and transoesophageal echocardiography), and should ideally be performed prior to the administration of antibiotics in order to prevent false negative culture results. Intravenous antibiotics targeting the responsible pathogen are usually needed for 4-6 weeks in the majority of patients.

Beyon RP, Bahl VK and Prendergast BD. Infective endocarditis. British Medical Journal. 2006;333:334-9

Cosgrove SE and Karchmer AW. Endocarditis. Medicine. 2005;33:66-72.

27) C: IV benzylpenicillin and gentamicin for at least 6 weeks

As well as surgery, involving the removal of gross vegetations and the replacement of the affected prosthetic valve, this patient will require a long course of intravenous antibiotics. Prosthetic valve endocarditis usually requires treatment with IV antibiotics for a duration of at least 6 weeks, whereas native valvular disease often requires 4-6 weeks of treatment.

In cases of confirmed streptococcal prosthetic valve endocarditis, IV benzylpenicillin and gentamicin is recommended for at least 6 weeks. If, however, the micro-organisms are fully sensitive to penicillin, then gentamicin can be stopped after 2 weeks. Streptococcal native valvular endocarditis would also require IV benzylpenicillin (with gentamicin if caused by less-sensitive streptococci), but for 4-6 weeks duration. In penicillin-allergic patients, or in highly-penicillin resistant streptococcal infections, the preferred antibiotic choice would be IV vancomycin with gentamicin.

The rationale for dual therapy of a cephalosporin (or a glycopeptide such as vancomycin) with aminoglycosides (namely gentamicin) is that these antibiotic pairs work synergistically. The cephalosporins and glycopeptides inhibit bacterial cell wall synthesis, which permit higher concentrations of gentamicin to enter the bacteria and inhibit ribosomal translocation and therefore protein synthesis.

Joint Formulary Committee (2011). British National Formulary. 61st edition. London: British Medical Association and Royal Pharmaceutical Society of Great Britain.

28) D: Hypomagnesaemia

Hypomagnesaemia causes a prolonged PR interval (>0.2 seconds).

Causes of a short PR interval include Lown Ganong Levine syndrome and Wolff Parkinson White syndrome which are both pre-excitation syndromes that are caused by conducting accessory pathways (called the bundle of James and Kent, respectively), which bypass the AV node and induce premature ventricular depolarisation. The ECG manifestation of LGL syndrome is a reduced PR interval occurring in the presence of a normal QRS complex, whilst WPW syndrome is further associated with a widened QRS complex due to slurring of the R wave (called the delta wave).

Pompe's and Fabry's disease are both glycogen storage disease who cardiac manifestations include the presence of shortened PR intervals.

European Resuscitation Council. Part 8: advanced challenges in resuscitation. Section 1: life-threatening electrolyte abnormalities. Resuscitation. 2000;46:253-9

MacKenzie R. Short PR interval. Journal of Insurance Medicine. 2005;37:145-52

29) A: Hypercalcaemia

Hypocalaemia, and not hypercalcaemia, is a well-recognised cause of QT prolongation. The importance of QT prolongation is underscored by the fact that it is a predisposing factor for Torsades de Pointes tachycardia. This is a characteristic polymorphic ventricular tachycardia with a twisting polarity, which can revert to sinus rhythm or degenerate into ventricular fibrillation potentially leading to sudden cardiac death.

Causes of QT prolongation are vast and include:

1) Genetic conditions – Romano-Ward and Jervell-Lange-Nielsen syndrome
2) Electrolyte disturbances – hypocalcaemia, hypomagnesaemia and hypokalaemia
3) Drugs – anti-arrhythmics, anti-depressants, antibiotics

Since the QT interval decreases with a rising heart rate, it can be corrected using the Bazett's formula or the Fridericia's formula, which involves dividing the QT interval by the square root or the cube root, respectively, of the R-R interval.

Abrams DJ, Perkin MA and Skinner JR. Long QT syndrome. 2010;340:b4815

30) D: In the Sudden Cardiac Death in Heart Failure Trial (SCD-HeFT) amiodarone was superior to placebo in improving survival among heart failure patients

Although Amiodarone is classified as a type III anti-arrhythmic in the Vaughan-Williams classification scheme (as it is an effective potassium channel blocker), it has a broad range of pharmacological effects that span blocking sodium channels, alpha- and beta-adrenoceptors and calcium channels. Additionally, amiodarone depresses sino-atrial nodal automaticity, increases the refractory period of the AV node and induces vasodilatation of the coronary and peripheral blood vessels.

The SCD-HeFT trial compared the effects of placebo, amiodarone and implantable cardioverter defibrillators (ICDs) in NYHA class II and III heart failure patients with an ejection fraction < 35%. The study showed that ICDs significantly improved mortality compared with amiodarone and placebo, but there were no survival benefits of amiodarone when compared with placebo.

Amiodarone raises serum digoxin levels by inhibiting its renal excretion, but it also raises the serum concentrations of many other drugs by reducing their metabolism via inhibition of several cytochrome p450 enzymes. For example, amiodarone can raise serum concentrations of warfarin, statins, calcium channel blockers, tacrolimus and flecainide among others.

Amiodarone is notorious for its vast range of side-effects, which is the reason why in 20-50% of patients, the drug must be discontinued. Side-effects of amiodarone include chemical pneumonitis, hypo- and hyperthyroidism, bradycardia, torsades de pointes, photosensitive skin discolouration, corneal deposition, cirrhosis and neurological disturbances (e.g. ataxia, tremor, peripheral neuropathy).

Bardy GH, Lee KL, Mark DB, Poole JE, Packer DL, Boineau R et al. Amiodarone or an implantable cardioverter-defibrillator for congestive heart failure. New England Journal of Medicine. 2005;352:225-37.

Van Erven L and Schalij MJ. Amiodarone: an effective antiarrhythmic drug with unusual side effect. Heart. 2010;96:1593-600

31) D: 2.5-5mg verapamil given intravenously over 2 minutes

The patient has a regular narrow-complex supraventricular tachycardia. Should carotid massage or valsalva manoeuvres (e.g. asking the patient to blow into a syringe) fail to terminate this arrhythmia, the next step is adenosine which, due to its very short half-life (10 seconds) must be given as a rapid IV bolus immediately followed by a saline flush in a large antecubital vein. However, severe asthma is an absolute contraindication for adenosine (as it causes bronchospasm) and beta blockers (which is an alternative treatment), leaving verapamil as the most appropriate option.

Option E represents treatment for ventricular tachycardia in stable patients.

If the patient had signs of adverse features (e.g. acute heart failure, myocardial ischaemia, syncope or shock), for any form of tachycardia with a pulse, then synchronised DC cardioversion would have been the most appropriate initial therapeutic strategy.

Pitcher D and Perkins G. Peri-arrest arrhythmias. Resuscitation Council Guidelines. 2010.

Venables P and Tomlinson DR. Supraventricular and ventricular arrhythmias: medical management. Medicine. 2010;38:515-21

32) B: The posterior descending artery represents a branch of the right coronary artery in up to 60% of individuals

The right and left coronary arteries originate in the ostia of the aortic sinuses, located immediately above the bases of the aortic valve cusps. The right coronary artery originates from the anterior sinus, the left from the left posterior sinus whilst the right posterior sinus is the non-coronary sinus.

Up to 90% of the general population have a 'right dominant heart,' which simply means that the posterior descending artery (PDA), running along the posterior interventricular groove towards the cardiac apex, is a branch of the right coronary artery in 90% of individuals. With left dominance, the PDA is supplied by the left coronary artery, usually the left circumflex.

The occurrence of new-onset AV conduction heart block in the context of a myocardial infarction should raise the suspicion of right coronary arterial involvement, as this coronary artery supplies the AV node in most patients (90%).

Thebesian veins, also known as the venae cordis minimae, represent small venous channels that originate within the myocardium, and penetrate through to the endocardium to drain into the closest chamber. They account for around 20-30% of all venous drainage, the remainder being predominantly via the coronary sinus.

Whitaker RH. Anatomy of the heart. Medicine. 2010; 38:333-35.

33) E: Simvastatin and furosemide

New-onset muscular pain in the setting of lipid lowering therapy should always be taken very seriously and consideration should be made to stopping the offending drug after reviewing the patient's drug history. With the exception of furosemide, all of the above drugs increase the risk of statin-induced myalgia, myopathy, myositis and rarely, in severe cases, rhabdomyolysis.

A serum creatine kinase (CK) level should be ordered as an abnormally high level may provide evidence of a myopathy. If the muscle pain is well tolerated by the patient, then statin therapy can continue providing that the CK level is less than 5 times the upper limit of the normal value. A urine dipstick may yield a false positive finding of haematuria due to myoglobin released from damaged skeletal muscle. Liver function tests would also be recommended in order to exclude evidence of liver damage in cases of statin toxicity. If serum transaminase levels exceed 3 times the upper limit of normal or if the patient has clinical symptoms or signs suggestive of liver damage, statin therapy should be stopped. In cases of rhabdomyolysis, there is significant risk of acute kidney injury, meaning that urea and electrolytes should also be checked.

Joint Formulary Committee (2011). British National Formulary. 61st edition. London: British Medical Association and Royal Pharmaceutical Society of Great Britain.

34) C: Digoxin toxicity due to hypokalaemia

The patient's symptoms are characteristic of digoxin toxicity. Elderly patients are particularly vulnerable to many adverse drug reactions owing to their reduced renal function reserves, which is especially noteworthy in this example as digoxin is predominantly excreted by the kidneys. Additionally, digoxin toxicity can be precipitated in the setting of normal serum digoxin levels if the patient is hypokalaemic which, in this example, was provoked by the combination of loop and thiazide diuretics (the effects of which may have been attenuated by ACE inhibitors).

One major way digoxin functions is by binding to the extracellular portion of the Na^+/K^+ ATPase, which would otherwise bind potassium ions. With low potassium levels, a greater proportion of the available digoxin is free to bind its target, thereby explaining why digoxin toxicity can be driven by hypokalaemia in the setting of normal serum digoxin levels.

35) A: 71%

Of all those people that have a disease, the proportion of those that are tested positive describes the sensitivity of the test. Whereas of all those people that do not have the disease, the proportion of those that are tested negative is the specificity.

On the other hand, of all those that test positive for a disease, the proportion that actually have the disease describes the positive predictive value. And of all those that test negative for a disease, the proportion without the disease describes the negative predictive value.

36) A: VVI

The first letter describes the chamber(s) that is paced. The second letter describes the chamber that is sensed. The third letter describes the response to the sensed information.

Bennett DH. Cardiac Arrhythmias: Practical Notes on Interpretation and Treatment. Seventh Edition. Hodder Arnold. 2006

Neurology Questions

1) A 67-year old man presents with a 2-hour history of sudden onset weakness, affecting his right arm and right leg, speech disturbance and a right-sided visual field defect.

Which of the following arteries is most likely to have been affected?

A. Basilar artery
B. Anterior cerebral artery
C. Lenticulostriate arteries
D. Middle cerebral artery
E. Posterior cerebral artery

2) Which of the following is the most common condition that mimics stroke?

A. Space occupying lesion
B. Hypoglycaemia
C. Sepsis
D. Seizure
E. Syncope

3) A 69-year old publican with a 40-pack year history of smoking wakes up at 08:25 feeling rather strange. As he tries to get out of bed, he realises that his right arm and leg are weak and that the right side of his vision is completely gone. When he calls his wife, they both notice that his speech is 'slurred.' She calls the ambulance, and they both arrive in Accident and Emergency at 09:05.

After taking a history and performing a quick examination, the on-call registrar arranges for an urgent CT scan of the head, which excludes an intracerebral haemorrhage at 09:30.

The patient's blood pressure is 168/92mmHg.

What is the next best plan of management?

A. Intravenous thrombolysis
B. Commence 300mg aspirin daily for 2 weeks
C. Contact neurosurgical registrar on-call for a possible decompressive craniectomy
D. Prescribe anti-hypertensives for prompt lowering of blood pressure
E. Prescribe prophylactic anticonvulsants

4) You are the junior doctor on-call and you see a 49-year old gentleman in the medical assessment unit. He has an 8-hour history of new-onset muscle weakness affecting his left leg and arm.

You discover that he has a 30-pack year history of smoking; he is a known hypertensive and suffers from poorly controlled type II diabetes. On examination, there is reduced power of the left upper and lower limbs (MRC grading 1/5 and 2/5, respectively). There are no other neurological deficits.

Which of the following is the most likely diagnosis?

A. Subarachnoid haemorrhage
B. Total Anterior Circulation Infarct (TACI)
C. Partial Anterior Circulation Infarct (PACI)
D. Posterior Circulation Infarct (POCI)
E. Lacunar Infarct (LACI)

5) Which of the following is the most common cause of subarachnoid haemorrhage?

A. Ruptured berry aneurysm
B. Trauma
C. Arterio-venous malformation
D. Pituitary apoplexy
E. Hypertension

6) You are a GP and an elderly male presents complaining of a rash on his nose. He states that he hasn't been feeling well over the past week as he has felt tired and lethargic.

On examination, the rash is localised to the left tip of the nose, is fairly well demarcated and is comprised of vesicles and pustules, some of which have crusted over.

How should you manage this patient?

A. Reassure the patient and tell him the rash will settle down.
B. Make an urgent referral to the hospital
C. Prescribe oral acyclovir 200mg fives times daily for five days
D. Give topical emollients and steroids, and tell the patient to come back if things don't settle
E. Perform a full eye examination and prescribe oral acyclovir 800mg five times daily for seven days.

7) You are a medical student undertaking a clinical placement in neurology and your consultant has been asked to see a patient who was admitted 1-week previously having sustained a stab injury to the back.

After examining the patient, he suspects a case of Brown-Sequard syndrome.

Which of the following constellation of neurological signs, with respect to the site of the lesion, is consistent with this syndrome?

A. Contralateral spastic paralysis, ipsilateral loss of fine touch, vibration and proprioception and contralateral loss of pain and temperature sensation
B. Contralateral spastic paralysis, contralateral loss of fine touch, vibration and proprioception and contralateral loss of pain and temperature sensation
C. Ipsilateral spastic paralysis, contralateral loss of fine touch, vibration and proprioception and contralateral loss of pain and temperature sensation
D. Ipsilateral spastic paralysis, ipsilateral loss of fine touch, vibration and proprioception and ipsilateral loss of pain and temperature sensation
E. Ipsilateral spastic paralysis, ipsilateral loss of fine touch, vibration and proprioception and contralateral loss of pain and temperature sensation

8) You are a medical student undertaking your neurology OSCE and you elicit an intriguing sign as you assess the horizontal smooth pursuit eye movements of a young lady.

You find that as the patient looks to her right, the right eye abducts, but the left eye fails to simultaneously adduct. Conjugate eye movements to the left are normal and no other neurological deficits are demonstrated.

Damage to which of the following neuroanatomical structures would account for this clinical finding?

A. Left occulomotor nerve
B. Left medial longitudinal fasciculus
C. Right medial longitudinal fasciculus
D. Left abducens nucleus
E. Left abducent nerve

9) You are the junior doctor on-call and you see a 68-year old gentleman in the medical assessment unit who presents with a 3-hour history of sudden, new-onset hoarseness of voice, difficulty swallowing, vertigo and drooping of the right eyelid.

He has a history of uncontrolled hypertension and is on 500mg BD metformin for type II diabetes. On examination, there is miosis and partial ptosis of the right eye, diminished pain and temperature sensation on the right side of the face and the left side of the body below the neck, ataxia affecting the right upper and lower limbs and a nystagmus. There are no other neurological deficits.

What is the most likely diagnosis?

A. Parinaud syndrome
B. Wallenberg's syndrome
C. Weber's syndrome
D. Collet-Sicard syndrome
E. Medial medullary syndrome

10) You are a house officer undertaking your neurology rotation and you see a 43-year old keen gardener who presents with a 3-month history of severe back pain and sciatica affecting her left leg.

A neurological examination is performed, which shows evidence of weakness of extension of the left big toe and diminished sensation over the dorsum of the left foot. Reflexes are preserved. Your registrar swiftly checks the MRI spine of this patient, which confirms his suspicion of a lateral disc prolapse.

Before you are able to scrutinise the scan further, he briskly closes the image and asks you which intervertebral disc is the culprit?

A. L1-L2
B. L2-L3
C. L3-L4
D. L4-L5
E. L5-S1

11) A 38-year old businessman presents to A and E with a 1-hour history of sudden-onset headache. The pain is excruciating, localised to the right side of the head and described 'as if someone was stabbing the back of my eye with a spear.' He also complains of a blocked nose and a watery red eye.

Clinical examination reveals a right partial ptosis, miosis with ipsilateral conjunctival injection and lacrimation. Temperature is 37.1 degrees, heart rate 110/min and respiratory rate 18/min.

Which of the following is the most likely diagnosis?

A. Migraine
B. Cluster headache
C. Acute angle-closure glaucoma
D. Meningitis
E. Subarachnoid haemorrhage

12) A 22-year old student is referred to a neurologist due to a history of recurrent headaches accompanied by nausea. The patient describes episodes where she experiences right-sided throbbing pain that usually lasts for 8-10 hours, during which she is unable to do anything and prefers to lie in a dark, quiet room. On further questioning, the patient is currently taking the combined oral contraceptive pill.

Which of the following is the most likely diagnosis?

A. Migraine
B. Tension headache
C. Subarachnoid haemorrhage
D. Meningitis
E. Venous Sinus Thrombosis

13) Which of the following is appropriate prophylaxis for regular tension headaches?

A. Paracetamol
B. Aspirin
C. Verapamil
D. Amitriptyline
E. Propranolol

14) A 57-year old carpenter presents to his GP with a 3-month history of facial pain. He describes severe episodes of lancinating pain of the left cheek, rated 10/10 in severity, but lasting for only a few seconds at a time. These episodes take place up to 10-15 times a day and have always been triggered by shaving.

Which of the following is the first-line management for this condition?

A. Phenytoin
B. Gabapentin
C. Amitriptyline
D. Lamotrigine
E. Carbamazepine

15) A 35-year old woman with a history of breast cancer is brought into accident and emergency with a 10-hour history of sudden-onset severe lower back pain and bilateral leg pain extending to below both knees.

Clinical examination reveals diminished ankle jerks bilaterally but preserved knee jerks, reduced sensation around the perianal region and a reduced anal tone on PR examination.

What is the most appropriate first-line investigation?

A. Urgent MRI of lumbosacral spine
B. Urgent radiograph of lumbosacral spine
C. Nerve conduction studies
D. CT spine
E. Bone profile

16) A 35-year old waiter is brought to the medical assessment unit with a 3-day history of worsening weakness of his lower limbs.

On examination, there is weakness of all movements of his lower limbs, especially affecting the hip flexors and knee extensors. Both knee and ankle jerk reflexes are absent.

On further questioning, the patient admits to a few episodes of diarrhoea 2 weeks previously.

Which of the following represents the most important investigation for this patient?

A. Nerve conduction studies
B. MRI of the spine
C. Serial monitoring of forced vital capacity
D. Lumbar puncture
E. CT head

17) A 33-year old nail technician sees her GP because of a 10-day history of slurred speech. She also states that over a year ago, she experienced blurring of vision affecting her right eye that lasted for about 2 weeks, though this has never quite fully recovered. On examination, the patient has a mildly ataxic gait, dysarthria, intention tremor, a right Marcus-Gunn pupil and visual acuity is 6/12 for the right eye and 6/6 for the left eye.

Which of the following is the most likely diagnosis?

   A. Multiple Sclerosis
   B. Amyotrophic lateral sclerosis
   C. Pseudobulbar palsy
   D. Ataxia-Telangiectasia
   E. Optic neuritis

18) Which of the following is NOT a clinical feature of optic neuritis?

   A. Marcus-Gunn pupil
   B. Red colour desaturation
   C. Pale disc on fundoscopy
   D. Pain on eye movement
   E. Holmes-Adie pupil

19) A patient known to have multiple sclerosis tells her neurologist that whenever she flexes her neck, she experiences electric-shocks shooting down her back and arms.

What is the name given to this clinical finding?

   A. Uhthoff's phenomenon
   B. Lhermitte's sign
   C. Pulfrich effect
   D. Levine's sign
   E. Hoffman's sign

20) Which of the following statements regarding the management of multiple sclerosis is incorrect?

A. There is a 1:1000 risk of developing a progressive multifocal leucoencephalopathy with Natalizumab
B. Mitoxantrone has a 1:300 risk of causing an acute leukaemia
C. Long term steroids play a key role in the management of multiple sclerosis
D. Baclofen can be used to relieve muscle spasticity
E. Beta interferons can reduce the frequency of relapses by approximately 30%

21) You are a medical student in the neurology outpatient's clinic with your consultant. You see a 65-year old ex-lorry driver who gives a 6-month history of recurrent falls without loss of consciousness and gradually progressive slowness in his movements.

On examination, the patient has a broad-based unsteady gait, slurred speech and limited volitional vertical eye movements, which appear preserved during the vestibular-ocular reflex. There is also evidence of increased rigidity on assessing muscle tone of the upper limbs. The consultant asks for your opinion.

Which of the following is the most likely diagnosis?

A. Friedreich's ataxia
B. Parkinson's disease
C. Cortico-basal degeneration
D. Steele-Richardson-Olszewski syndrome
E. Shy-Drager syndrome

22) Which of the following is NOT a sign of Parkinson's disease?

A. Postural instability
B. Bradykinesia
C. Pill-rolling tremor of 5-10 Hz
D. Festinating gait
E. Camptocormia

23) What is the mechanism of action of the anti-Parkinsonian drug entacapone?

    A. Dopamine receptor agonist
    B. COMT inhibitor
    C. Peripheral DOPA decarboxylase inhibitor
    D. MAO-A inhibitor
    E. MAO-B inhibitor

24) A 68-year old retired businessman presents with a 10-month history of resting tremor, predominantly affecting the right hand. The patient also admits to feeling depressed recently ever since his wife left him 1 month ago.

On examination, the patient has evidence of bradykinesia, rigidity of both upper limbs and inspection of the gait reveals a festinating gait with reduced arm swing. Standing blood pressure is 110/82 mmHg, whilst lying blood pressure is 86/68 mmHg.

What is the most likely diagnosis?

    A. Lewy-body dementia
    B. Parkinson's disease
    C. Cortico-basal degeneration
    D. Progressive Supranuclear Palsy
    E. Shy-Drager syndrome

25) A 19-year old girl is referred to a neurologist after experiencing several episodes of loss of consciousness. Her parents state that when these episodes occur, their daughter collapses to the ground, shakes violently for about a minute and becomes incontinent of urine. After she regains consciousness, she appears drowsy and confused for several hours and often complains of a sore tongue.

The neurologist makes a diagnosis and decides to instigate treatment after a discussion with the patient and her family.

Which of the following is the most appropriate first-line pharmacological treatment?

A. Lamotrigine
B. Carbamazepine
C. Sodium Valproate
D. Topiramate
E. Ethosuximide

26) The parents bring their 8-year old boy to see their GP as they are worried about their son's behaviour. They describe periods where their son stops in mid-sentence, stares blankly ahead and remains unresponsive for nearly 10 seconds before he completes the sentence as if nothing had happened.

This occurs up to 50 times a day.

What is the most likely diagnosis?

A. Temporal lobe epilepsy
B. Absence epilepsy
C. Juvenile myoclonic epilepsy
D. Lennox-Gastaut syndrome
E. West syndrome

27) Which of the following regarding Juvenile Myoclonic Epilepsy (JME) is FALSE?

A. Myoclonic jerks is seen in 100% of cases and forms an essential part of the definition
B. Generalised tonic-clonic seizures occur in up to 90-95% of patients with JME
C. Absence seizures occur in around 5% of patients with JME
D. The drug of choice is sodium valproate
E. Lifelong anticonvulsant treatment is highly recommended

28) A 42-year old lorry driver was recently diagnosed with temporal lobe epilepsy by his neurologist.

According to DVLA regulations, how long must he remain seizure-free without anticonvulsants before he can reapply for his HGV license?

A. 6 months
B. 1 year
C. 3 years
D. 5 years
E. 10 years

29) A GP takes a history from a 32-year old teacher who presents with a 4-month history of muscle weakness and double vision worse towards the end of the day.

On examination, tendon reflexes are preserved, but after abducting and adducting the shoulders repeatedly, shoulder weakness becomes substantially more pronounced.

Which of the following is FALSE about this condition?

A. It is caused by autoantibodies targeting nicotinic acetylcholine receptors or muscle specific tyrosine kinase
B. The early onset form of the condition affects women more commonly than men
C. The Tensilon test represents a useful diagnostic tool
D. Single fibre electromyography may show increased jitter
E. Is associated with thymoma in 60% of cases

30) A 40-year old plumber sees his doctor as he is concerned that both his hands have become gradually weaker over the past year.

On examination there is thenar and hypothenar muscle wasting bilaterally, and clawing of both hands. The GP completes a full neurological examination and discovers a selective loss of pain and temperature sensation bilaterally, affecting the neck, both arms and down to the upper part of the trunk. No other neurological signs are elicited.

Which of the following is the most likely diagnosis?

A. Cervical spondylotic myelopathy
B. Syringomyelia
C. Brown-Sequard syndrome
D. Syringobulbia
E. Tabes dorsalis

31) A previously fit and well 42-year old accountant develops sudden-onset 'thunderclap' frontal headache accompanied by vomiting. He is seen by a physician in the emergency department 1-hour later.

On examination, the patient's right eye is deviated inferiorly and laterally, and is associated with an ipsilateral ptosis and pupillary dilation. The patient also complains of some visual loss.

A CT head shows a heterogeneous opacification within the suprasellar cistern.

Which of the following is the single most important acute medical management?

A. High-dose corticosteroids
B. Oral nimodipine
C. Intravenous infusion of mannitol
D. Broad-spectrum antibiotics
E. Vasopressors and inotropic support

32) A 46-year old chronic alcoholic is admitted with a head injury and initially appears unresponsive to voice. The patient has a patent airway, is breathing spontaneously and has a pulse. As a doctor tries to secure an IV line, the patient opens both his eyes, mumbles some sounds and uses his opposite hand to push the doctor away.

What is the patient's Glasgow Coma Score (GCS)?

A. 6
B. 7
C. 8
D. 9
E. 10

33) After taking a history from a middle-aged lady complaining of burning pain of her right lower limb, the neurologist makes a diagnosis of meralgia paraesthetica.

Which nerve is affected?

A. Lateral cutaneous nerve of the thigh
B. Sural nerve
C. Femoral nerve
D. Sciatic nerve
E. Obturator nerve

34) All of the following muscles are innervated by the median nerve EXCEPT for:

A. Lateral two lumbricals
B. Opponens pollicis
C. Adductor pollicis
D. Abductor pollicis brevis
E. Flexor pollicis brevis

35) Which type of visual field defect is most likely to be seen following damage to Meyer's loop?

A. Contralateral homonymous hemianopia
B. Contralateral homonymous superior quadrantanopia
C. Contralateral homonymous inferior quadrantanopia
D. Ipsilateral homonymous superior quadrantanopia
E. Ipsilateral homonymous inferior quadrantanopia

36) Which of the following concerning motor neurone disease (MND) is FALSE?

A. Mean age of onset in the UK is in the sixth decade
B. It is a rare condition with an incidence of around 2/100,000 per year
C. Riluzole can prolong life in MND patients by 3-4 months on average
D. The familial form accounts for nearly 5% of cases of MND
E. The most common variant of MND is primary lateral sclerosis

37) A 16-year old male student is admitted to hospital with a 24-history of headache, neck stiffness, photophobia and vomiting. The on-call consultant physician considers a lumbar puncture as part of the management plan.

Which of the following is NOT a contraindication for this procedure?

A. Papilloedema
B. Dilated pupils poorly reactive to light
C. New focal neurological deficits
D. GCS dropping from 15 to 12
E. Platelet count of 110 x 10^9/litre

38) You are the junior doctor on-call and you see a 53-year old male accompanied by his wife in the medical assessment unit.

He has a 10-day history of progressively worsening headache, lethargy, nausea and vomiting. As you clerk him, you notice he appears quite confused and drowsy.

Heart rate is 120/min, respiratory rate 20/min and temperature is 38.9°C.

Before you are able to examine him further, he develops a tonic-clonic seizure lasting for a few minutes, which you manage appropriately. After instigating standard treatment for sepsis, your registrar decides to arrange an MRI brain scan. This reveals areas of hyperintensity localised to the anterior portions of the left temporal lobe.

What is the most likely diagnosis?

A. Toxoplasmosis
B. Herpes simplex encephalitis
C. Progressive multifocal leucoencephalopathy
D. Autoimmune encephalitis
E. Cryptococcal encephalitis

39) Following a traumatic injury, a 23-year old male develops a left-sided wrist drop.

On examination, there is weakness of forearm supination, weakness of extension at the wrist and metacarpophalangeal joints, an intact triceps jerk reflex and reduced sensation in the region of the left first dorsal interosseous only.

Where is the lesion?

A. Radial nerve – spiral groove
B. Radial nerve - wrist
C. Radial nerve - axilla
D. Radial nerve - forearm
E. C5-T1 nerve roots

40) A 72-year old gentleman presents to his GP with a 3-day history of right-sided facial weakness. On examination, right-sided facial drooping is evident with a lack of forehead wrinkling on the same side when raising the eyebrows. The GP also notices a rash in the right ear.

What is the most likely diagnosis?

A. Ramsay-Hunt syndrome
B. Bell's palsy
C. Lyme disease
D. Stroke
E. Brain tumour

Neurology Answers

1) D: Middle cerebral artery

A rudimentary understanding of brain anatomy and the corresponding vascular territories will enable one to understand the array of clinical manifestations that can arise in different stroke syndromes (see answer 4 for further details).

2) D: Seizure

There are multiple stroke mimics, which must always be considered in the differential diagnosis of someone presenting with focal neurological features. The muscle weakness that occurs in the post-ictal phase of tonic-clonic seizures (Todd's palsy) can often be confused with stroke if the ictal phase was un-witnessed.

McArthur KS, Quinn TJ, Dawson J and Walters MR. Diagnosis and management of transient ischaemic attack and ischaemic stroke in the acute phase. British Medical Journal. 2011; 342:d1938

Hand PJ, Kwan J, Lindley RI, Dennis MS, Wardlaw JM. Distinguishing between stroke and mimic at the bedside: the Brain Attack Study. Stroke 2006;37:769-75.

3) B: Commence 300mg aspirin daily for 2 weeks

Once a cerebral bleed has been excluded, and providing there are no contraindications, intravenous thrombolysis should be started within 3 hours of the onset of an ischaemic stroke (IV alteplase is licensed for use within 3 hours, but the evidence suggests benefits for up to 4.5 hours after the onset of an ischaemic stroke). This patient, however, is not eligible for thrombolysis because, as he woke up with symptoms, it is not exactly clear when his neurological deficit began.

A decompressive craniectomy is only considered in patients younger than 60 years and providing a CT head reveals substantial cerebral oedema causing a mass effect, which isn't the case in this scenario.

Although management of hypertension forms an important aspect of secondary stroke prevention, studies have shown that in the acute phase active antihypertensive measures may in fact increase the risk of harm to patients.

Even though stroke represents the most common cause of new-onset seizures in the elderly population, anti-convulsant prophylaxis immediately following stroke is not recommended.

Following 2 weeks of aspirin antiplatelet therapy, clopidogrel is commenced at a dose of 75mg/day lifelong.

Sandset EC, Bath PM, Boysen G, Jatuzis D, Kõrv J, Lüders S, et al. The angiotensin-receptor blocker candesartan for treatment of acute stroke (SCAST): a randomised, placebo-controlled, double-blind trial. Lancet 2011;337:741-50.

Reckless IP and Buchan AM. Stroke: management and prevention. Medicine 2008;36; 592-600.

McArthur KS, Quinn TJ, Dawson J and Walters MR. Diagnosis and management of transient ischaemic attack and ischaemic stroke in the acute phase. British Medical Journal. 2011; 342:d1938

4) E: Lacunar Infarct (LACI)

This patient had an ischaemic stroke (the absence of headache makes subarachnoid haemorrhage highly unlikely). The Bamford classification offers a useful tool for subclassifying ischaemic strokes into clinical syndromes of prognostic value. These syndromes are divided according to the compromised vascular territory and thus spatial region of the brain that has infarcted (see below):

Total Anterior Circulation Infarct (TACI, Proximal middle cerebral artery (MCA)) – All 3 of the following:

a) New higher cortical dysfunction (e.g. dysphasia, visuospatial disorder, dyscalculia)
b) Homonymous hemianopia
c) Contralateral sensory and/or motor deficit affecting at least 2/3 of the face, arms and legs.

====

Partial Anterior Circulation Infarct (PACI, Distal branch of MCA) - Any of the following:

a) Two out of three components of TACI
b) Isolated higher cortical dysfunction
c) Motor or sensory deficit confined to a single limb, face or hand (not whole arm)

Posterior Circulation Infarct (POCI, Vertebrobasilar territory) - Any of the following:

a) Ipsilateral cranial nerve palsy with contralateral motor and/or sensory deficit
b) Bilateral motor and/or sensory deficit
c) Internuclear ophthalmoplegia
d) Isolated cerebellar dysfunction
e) Isolated homonymous hemianopia

LACI (Deep perforating arteries) –Any of the following (all involving at least 2/3 of the face, arms and legs):

a) Pure motor stroke
b) Pure sensory stroke
c) Sensorimotor stroke
d) Ataxic hemiparesis

Bamford J, Sandercock P, Dennis M, Warlow C, Burn J. Classification and natural history of clinically identifiable subtypes of cerebral infarction. Lancet 1991;337:1521-6.

5) **B: Trauma**

Although a ruptured berry aneurysm is a frequently cited cause of a subarachnoid haemorrhage, trauma by far constitutes the most common aetiology.

6) **E: Perform a full eye examination and prescribe oral acyclovir 800mg five times daily for seven days.**

This is a case of shingles affecting the ophthalmic division of the trigeminal nerve. Shingles is caused by the reactivation of the varicella-zoster virus (the same virus that causes chicken pox), from its dormant state in the dorsal root ganglion of the affected nerve. During reactivation, the virus migrates to the skin innervated by the corresponding nerve root, resulting in a skin lesion characteristically localised to a dermatomal distribution. Prior to shingles visibly manifesting itself on the skin, patients often experience vague prodromal flu-like symptoms lasting for up to one week, encompassing a low-grade fever, malaise and fatigue. The skin lesions then appear, within the affected dermatome, first as macules sequentially progressing to papules, vesicles and pustules, which finally crust over and clear over several weeks (though scarring may be apparent in some cases). Shingles are painful (classically referred to as 'a belt of roses from hell') and patients often experience neuropathic-type pain such as shooting or burning sensations, which may persist even after clearance of the skin lesion as a post-herpetic neuralgia.

This particular case example is not a common presentation of shingles, but it's designed to illustrate an important concept, namely Hutchinson's sign. The skin lesion is located at the tip of the nose, which is specifically innervated by the nasociliary branch of the ophthalmic division of the trigeminal nerve. The same branch also innervates the ipsilateral cornea. Therefore, if shingles presents itself on the tip of the nose, it suggests a significant probability of impending ocular involvement, potentially resulting in a keratitis and subsequent corneal scarring. This explains the necessity of performing a full eye examination and ophthalmological referral if necessary. Anti-viral therapy is also required to reduce the risk of complications from shingles but at a higher dose (800mg fives times daily for seven days) than in uncomplicated herpes-simplex infections (200mg fives times daily for five days).

Shaikh S and Ta CN. Evaluation and management of herpes zoster ophthalmicus. American Family Physician. 2002; 66:1723-30.

7) **E: Ipsilateral spastic paralysis, ipsilateral loss of fine touch, vibration and proprioception and contralateral loss of pain and temperature sensation**

Brown-sequard syndrome is a rare condition that classically occurs following hemisection of the spinal cord; the most common aetiology being blunt or penetrating injuries. However, anything that damages or compresses one half of the spinal cord can result in the syndrome, including malignancies, multiple sclerosis, spinal cord infarction and bleeding (e.g. an epidural haematoma).

Answering this question requires a good working knowledge of the anatomy of 3 of the major neural pathways running in the spinal cord:

a) The dorsal column-medial lemniscus pathway, which is responsible for transmitting sensory information spanning fine discriminative touch, vibratory and joint position sense (proprioception).

b) The spinothalamic tract, which is responsible for transmitting pain and temperature sensation.

c) Corticospinal tract, which is responsible for motor function.

The key to understanding Brown-Sequard syndrome requires knowledge of the fact that spinothalamic tract neurons decussate (i.e. cross the midline) at roughly the same level as the corresponding primary sensory afferents carrying pain and temperature information to these neurons.

However, in the case of the dorsal column-medial lemniscus pathway and the corticospinal tract, decussation of the neurons occurs at the level of the medulla. Therefore a lesion affecting half the cord would damage dorsal column fibres carrying ipsilateral sensory information, corticospinal tract conveying ipsilateral motor information and spinothalamic fibres carrying contralateral sensory information.

Nolte J. The Human Brain: An Introduction to Its Functional Anatomy, Fifth Edition. Mosby. 2002

8) B: Left medial longitudinal fasciculus

This is a case of internuclear ophthalmoplegia, and although unlikely to come up in neurology OSCEs for finals (unless the examiner is very mean!), it illustrates the elegance of pinpointing the precise location of a lesion in the central nervous system by applying relevant neuroanatomical knowledge to a clinical context. The medial longitudinal fasciculus (MLF) is a tract of nerve fibres in the brainstem that connects the abducens nucleus (in the caudal pons) to the contralateral, rostrally located occulomotor nucleus in the midbrain (specifically the part that comprises neurons innervating the medial rectus muscle). When you look to your right, the right abducens nucleus (and consequently abducent nerve) is activated, causing right eye abduction. At the same time, another group of neurons arising in the right abducens nucleus, which decussate at that level to form the left MLF, are activated. This leads to activation of left medial rectus motor neurons and consequently adduction of the left eye when looking to the right, under normal circumstances. If there is a lesion in the MLF, then such conjugate eye movements are no longer possible.

The fact that the patient has no other neurological findings on eye examination excludes damage to the occulomotor nerve.

Nolte J. The Human Brain: An Introduction to Its Functional Anatomy, Fifth Edition. Mosby. 2002

9) B: Wallenberg's syndrome

Given the sudden onset of the neurological symptoms as well as the risk factors of hypertension and type II diabetes, this patient is most likely to have had a stroke. However, the unusual constellation of clinical findings should raise the possibility of a small infarct in the brainstem. In this case, the posterior-inferior cerebellar artery, which supplies the lateral part of the medulla, represents the affected vascular territory resulting in the lateral medullary syndrome (Wallenberg's syndrome). The lateral medulla carries several important neural structures, and damage to it can explain the patient's presenting symptoms and signs. Damage to the:

a) Nucleus ambiguus, which sends lower motor neurons via the glossopharyngeal nerve (cranial nerve IX) innervating pharyngeal and laryngeal musculature, explains the new onset dysphagia and dysphonia.

b) Central sympathetic nerve fibres (which descend to synapse with sympathetic preganglionic neurons) explain the new onset Horner's syndrome.

c) Spinal trigeminal tract and nucleus carrying sensory afferents from the ipsilateral side of the face explains the loss of pain and temperature sensation on the same side.

d) Spinothalamic tract explains the loss of pain and temperature sensation on the contralateral side of the body (recall that at the level of the medulla, all spinothalamic nerve fibres throughout the cord have already decussated).

e) Vestibular nuclei explains the vertigo

f) Inferior cerebellar peduncle (carrying neurons to the cerebellum) explains the ataxia and nystagmus.

Nolte J. The Human Brain: An Introduction to Its Functional Anatomy, Fifth Edition. Mosby. 2002

10) D: L4-L5

Knowledge of dermatomes and myotomes are frequently assessed in both written examinations and OSCEs. This question requires you to identify not only which nerve root the prolapsed disc has compressed but also which disc is involved. Big toe extension specifically tests L5, whilst the L5 dermatome covers the dorsum of the foot. Lower limb reflexes are preserved in this patient since knee jerk is L3 and L4, whilst ankle jerk tests predominantly S1. To answer this question correctly, it is necessary to understand that when a disc prolapses, the spinal nerve root that is compressed is the one that lies *below* the disc.

11) B: Cluster headache

The patient describes a good history of cluster headache. The clinical features that reliably differentiate cluster headache from other types of headache disorders are the combination of the characteristic type of pain experienced, the accompanying cranial autonomic manifestations and the cyclical nature of cluster headaches (episodes are commonly grouped in clusters, hence the name). Cluster headaches are highly excruciating, classically lasting 15-180 minutes per episode with a frequency of 1 every other day to 8 times per day. Pain is most commonly unilateral, felt behind the eye but may be felt temporally or over the maxilla. Cranial autonomic features localised *ipsilateral to the headache* include nasal congestion/rhinorrhoea, lacrimation, conjunctival injection, partial ptosis with miosis (Horner's syndrome) and forehead/facial sweating (though not all features need to be present at the same time).

Patients with cluster headache often appear restless or agitated during attacks in contrast to patients with migraine. Acute angle-closure glaucoma, an important cause of the acutely painful red eye, is accompanied by reduced visual acuity, a fixed mid-dilated pupil and corneal clouding.

Features of meningism (headache, photophobia and neck stiffness) would predominate in cases of meningitis and subarachnoid haemorrhage. Additionally, the absence of pyrexia makes meningitis less likely.

Nesbitt A.D. and Goadsby, PJ. Cluster Headache. British Medical Journal. 2012;344: 37-42.

Headache Classification Committee of the International Headache Society. The international classification of headache disorders (second edition). Cephalalgia 2004: 24 (suppl 1): 1-160.

12) A: Migraine

Migraine attacks are gradual in onset, characteristically unilateral (but not always), throbbing in nature, lasting 4-72 hours and accompanied by nausea or vomiting. 'Preferring to lie in a dark, quiet room' is code for 'this patient has photophobia and phonophobia, respectively,' both symptoms of which are commonly seen in this condition. Furthermore, the contraceptive pill is a well-recognised risk factor for migraines. Classical migraines are preceded by auras lasting minutes to an hour, though these only comprise approximately 20% of migraines. Such auras may be visual and include zig-zag lines, fortification spectra, scintillating lines/dots or scotomata. Auras may also be haptic in nature, characteristically a paraesthesia spreading like a wave from the fingers to the face. Importantly, an aura may actually mimic a transient ischaemic attack and could manifest itself as a temporary hemianopia, hemiplegia or dysphasia.

The recurrent history of the headache in this patient makes subarachnoid haemorrhage, venous sinus thrombosis and meningitis less likely than the other options. A subarachnoid haemorrhage typically presents with sudden onset "thunderclap headache," usually associated with meningism and vomiting. In a convincing history with such a sudden onset, severe headache, a CT head is mandatory, although it cannot exclude a small subarachnoid bleed, as in 5-10% of cases, false negatives occur, in which case a lumbar puncture is necessary. This should be performed promptly, but a minimum of 12 hours should elapse after onset of headache to allow for the greatest diagnostic yield, looking in particular for CSF xanthochromia. In delayed presentations, an LP can be performed for up to 2 weeks after headache onset. A negative LP can reliably exclude a subarachnoid haemorrhage. Venous sinus thrombosis can present in a similar manner to a subarachnoid bleed, so in patients where there is a high index of suspicion (for example, convincing history, LP negative for xanthochromia, pro-thrombotic risk factors), a CT or MR venogram should be considered.

Cluster headaches have been previously described. Tension headaches are very common, often less disabling than migraines, non-pulsatile in nature and feel like a tight band around the head, which is not the case in this patient.

Scottish Intercollegiate Guidelines Network. Diagnosis and management of headache in adults.2008.

13) D: Amitriptyline

Paracetamol or aspirin represent appropriate *acute* treatments for tension headaches. However, when headaches become a regular phenomenon, prophylactic measures should be taken in order to improve patient quality of life. SIGN guidelines recommend amitriptyline as the appropriate prophylaxis for regular tension headaches. Verapamil and propranolol represent prophylactic treatments for cluster headache and migraine, respectively.

Scottish Intercollegiate Guidelines Network. Diagnosis and management of headache in adults. 2008.

14) E: Carbamazepine

Although all of the drugs on the list are effective against neuropathic pain, carbamazepine is the first-line treatment for trigeminal neuralgia.

Bennetto L, Patel NK and Fuller G. Trigeminal neuralgia and its management. British Medical Journal. 2007;334:201

15) A: Urgent MRI of lumbosacral spine

This patient has cauda equina syndrome, which is most commonly caused by a centrally prolapsing disc compressing the cauda equina usually at the L4/5 or L5/S1 level (recall that the spinal cord terminates between L1 and L2, below which the cauda equina resides). This syndrome is a clinical emergency, requiring urgent MRI of the lumbosacral spine in order to confirm the diagnosis. The history of breast cancer raises the possibility of a bony metastatic lesion(s) in the vertebrae, which could alternatively account for this patient's symptoms and signs.

Treatment would depend on aetiology. In disc prolapses, this would involve prompt decompression performed by the neurosurgeons, ideally within 24 hours of symptom onset to maximise the chances of saving sphincter function. In cauda equina syndrome caused by bony metastases, this would usually require urgent radiotherapy.

Delays in diagnosis and management of this condition account for great patient morbidity and high litigation rates.

Cauda equina syndrome is characterised by the S's: Sciatica, Saddle anaesthesia, Sphincter disturbances and/or loss of Sexual function. (Note that to qualify as sciatica, lower back pain must radiate to below the knees). Sphincter disturbances include urinary retention, overflow incontinence and constipation or faecal incontinence. Patients with cauda equina syndrome will often have flaccid lower limb weakness and diminished reflexes at the affected level as the motor deficit is due to a lower motor neuron lesion.

Cord compression is another medical emergency, which can also be caused by disc prolapses and bony metastases (most common causes cited in exams). Although upper motor neuron signs would be expected, in the acute phase of the pathology lower motor neuron signs are paradoxically present (the so-called phase of spinal shock). With time, upper motor neuron signs then predominate.

Lavy C, James A, Wilson-MacDonald J and Fairbank J. Cauda equina syndrome. British Medical Journal. 2009;338: 881-884.

16) C: Serial monitoring of forced vital capacity

This patient is most likely to have Guillain-Barre syndrome. This often presents with a rapidly progressive history of symmetrically ascending motor polyneuropathy, causing weakness that may be worse in the proximal muscles of the lower limbs, but may also affect distal muscles.

The aetiology is one of demyelination of lower motor neurons secondary, in around 75% of cases, to infection by a group of microorganisms including Campylobacter Jejuni (as in this scenario), Epstein-Barr virus, Influenza, Cytomegalovirus, HIV or Mycoplasma (the mechanism is thought to be molecular mimicry). Therefore, take heed of any preceeding infections from the history, usually 2-4 weeks previously, and especially those affecting the respiratory or gastrointestinal tract.

Later in the acute course of the disease, patients commonly develop weakness of the upper limbs, truncal muscles, facial, bulbar and respiratory muscles. Although a rare condition (incidence is around 1.2-1.6/100,000 per year), Guillain-Barre syndrome has a 10% mortality rate mostly due to respiratory muscle involvement; patients can develop respiratory failure, require ventilation in ITU, during which they are bedridden for protracted time periods, increasing the risk of hospital-acquired pneumonias and pulmonary embolism, which represent some of the most common causes of death in this condition. Therefore it is imperative to identify respiratory muscle weakness early in the course of the disease, through regular lung function tests, in order to promptly escalate appropriate cases to ITU.

Although nerve conduction studies and lumbar punctures (which characteristically show an albumino-cytological dissociation) can be useful in confirming the diagnosis, these come secondary in importance to lung function tests.

Winer JB. Guillain-Barre syndrome. British Medical Journal. 2008;337: 227-231.

17) A: Multiple Sclerosis

Multiple sclerosis (MS) is a chronic inflammatory, demyelinating condition of the central nervous system. The pathology is not restricted to demyelination of white matter, as was traditionally believed, but also encompasses axonal loss, which is thought to account for the permanent neurological sequelae inherent to most MS patients particularly during the later stages of the illness. It is more common in women (F:M is approximately 3:1) and has a predilection for affecting young people (mean age of onset is around 30 years). The epidemiology of MS is interesting in that the prevalence seems to rise the further away from the equator you move, although the exact aetiology remains unclear.

Several subtypes of MS exist, the most common of which is the *relapsing-remitting* form, which accounts for 80% of cases. In this clinical subtype, patients experience symptomatic episodes during relapses lasting for days to weeks and less commonly months, after which they recover completely or partially recover with some persisting neurological deficits. Between relapses, there is a lack of disease progression. During the first 10 years of their illness, however, approximately half of patients with relapsing-remitting MS develop *secondary progressive MS*, whereby periods of remission become replaced by a gradual deterioration in neurology and consequently disability. Nearly 10-15% of MS patients have the *primary progressive* phenotype where there is gradual, progressive deterioration in clinical symptoms from the outset of the disease. Other subtypes exist, such as *benign*, *malignant* and *progressive-relapsing MS*, though these are less common.

The diagnosis of MS is mainly clinical, requiring evidence of CNS lesions disseminated in space (i.e. more than 1 part of the CNS) and time (i.e. clinical symptoms or signs occurring on more than 1 occasion). This patient has cerebellar symptoms and signs, and a history of optic neuritis, which are common clinical manifestations. Other clinical features include fatigue and depression (very common), transverse myelitis (less common), sensory disturbances (sensory loss, paraesthesias or dysaesthesia) and sexual dysfunction. Clinical findings on eye examination include that of a Marcus Gunn pupil – where that pupil appears to dilate whilst a torch swings from the opposite eye to the affected one – this is known as a relative afferent pupillary defect (see answer 18 for further information).

Diagnostic investigations include MRI (which characteristically show periventricular or subcortical white matter plaques, if the brain is affected; although clinical and neuroimaging findings do not necessarily correlate), lumbar puncture (which may show oligoclonal bands in CSF that are not present in the serum; paired serum and CSF samples should therefore be taken) and measuring any delays in sensory-evoked potentials.

National Institute for Health and Clinical Excellence. 2003. Multiple Sclerosis: National clinical guidelines for diagnosis and management in primary and secondary care [CG8]. London: National Institute for Health and Clinical Excellence

18) E. Holmes-Adie pupil

Marcus-Gunn pupil is the eponymous equivalent of a relative afferent pupillary defect (RAPD), commonly seen in optic neuritis, and elicited in the swinging flashlight test. This test involves shining light on one eye, then swinging the flashlight to the opposite eye and briskly swinging the light back to the original eye; if the pupil that was shone first undergoes a relative dilation when it's shone for the second time, then that pupil is a Marcus-Gunn pupil and the test is positive. In order to understand the test further, let us analyse the neuroscientific basis underpinning the test.

Shining light on an eye will induce constriction of the ipsilateral pupil, due to activation of the direct reflex pathway, and contralateral pupil due to activation of the consensual reflex pathway. Both pathways have as their afferent and efferent arcs the optic and oculomotor nerves, respectively (see pathways below):

Direct pathway: Shining light on left eye → left optic nerve afferents → central connections* → left oculomotor nerve efferents → constriction of left pupil

Consensual pathway: Shining light on left eye → left optic nerve afferents → central connections* → right oculomotor nerve efferents → constriction of right pupil

central connections involve neural connections with the pretectal area (located between the thalamus above and the midbrain below) that send neurons to the Edinger-Westphal nuclei bilaterally, which provide parasympathetic efferents that reach the pupils via the oculomotor nerves.

If there is a left-sided optic neuritis, which would slow down nerve conduction velocities in the left optic nerve, shining light on the left eye would yield a relatively weak activation of the direct pathway, but would nonetheless induce some constriction of the left pupil. However, when shining light on the right eye (as the pen-torch is swung from the left to the right), the compromised left optic nerve is bypassed, and assuming a normally functioning right optic nerve (and occulomotor nerves bilaterally), activation of the consensual reflex pathway would be relatively stronger. Consequently, the consensual reflex pathway would yield greater constriction of the left pupil than the direct reflex pathway. This means that when the pen-torch is swung back to the left eye, and reverting to the weaker direct pathway, a relative pupillary dilation occurs as there is *less pupillary constriction*. Thus, the left pupil is the Marcus-Gunn pupil in this example.

A Holmes- Adie pupil can be a normal variant, but can also represent damage to the parasympathetic pupillary efferent fibres, resulting in a dilated myotonic pupil poorly reactive to light. Holmes-Adie syndrome is the association of a Holmes-Adie pupil with areflexia.

Nolte J. The Human Brain: An Introduction to Its Functional Anatomy, Fifth Edition. Mosby. 2002.

19) **B: Lhermitte's sign**

Lhermitte's sign is not quite pathognomonic of multiple sclerosis since it can also occur in cervical myelopathies.

Uhthoff's phenomenon describes the situation where symptoms experienced by MS patients become exacerbated by any activity that raises the core body temperature (e.g. exercise, hot baths etc).

The Pulfrich effect can occur in optic neuritis and describes the perception of straight trajectories appearing distorted owing to differential latencies in conduction velocities between the normal and compromised optic nerves.

Hoffman's sign is a sign of upper motor neuron disease and is positive when flicking a patient's finger results in a flexion motion of the ipsilateral thumb.

Levine's sign is not neurological and is classically suggestive of ischaemic cardiac chest pain when a patient places a fist over their chest.

20) C: Long-term steroids play a key role in the management of multiple sclerosis '

Short bursts of steroid therapy (e.g. 500mg-1g methylprednisolone IV for 3-5 days), not long term steroids, are recommended for patients suffering from symptomatic relapses sufficient to cause distress or impair activities of daily living. Unlike disease modifying therapy (e.g. beta-interferons, Glatiramer acetate, mitoxantrone and certain monoclonal immunoglobulins), steroids do not reduce the frequency of relapses or delay disability, but rather facilitate recovery of symptoms during a relapse.

National Institute for Health and Clinical Excellence. 2003. Multiple Sclerosis: National clinical guidelines for diagnosis and management in primary and secondary care [CG8]. London: National Institute for Health and Clinical Excellence

21) D: Steele-Richardson-Olszewski syndrome

The patient has Steele-Richardson-Olszewski syndrome, also known as Progressive Supranuclear Palsy (PSP), which represents one of the Parkinsons-Plus syndromes. Patients with PSP have postural instability and are liable to recurrent falls early in the clinical course of the illness. Some clinical features of PSP overlap with cerebellar disease, such as the broad-based unsteady gait and dysarthria, although patients with cerebellar disease would be expected to have hypotonia and not rigidity.

The key to differentiating PSP from Parkinson's disease is the combination of supranuclear vertical gaze palsy, recurrent falls and rigidity that is more prominent in the trunk than the limbs and arises in the absence of tremor (tremor is unusual in PSP) in PSP. The vertical gaze palsy is supranuclear as the lesion lies rostral to the occulomotor nucleus, so that volitional vertical eye movements are impaired (neural connections between the cerebral cortex and occulomotor nucleus are compromised), but since local reflex connections are still preserved, vertical eye movements can be produced using the doll's head manoeuvre (vestibular-ocular reflex).

Friedrich's ataxia is a hereditary condition associated with a cerebellar syndrome, diabetes mellitus, a cardiomyopathy and symptoms would not present with such a short onset as it is usually diagnosed in adolescence.

http://www.ninds.nih.gov/disorders/psp/detail_psp.htm

Jankovic J. Parkinson's disease: clinical features and diagnosis. Journal of Neurology, Neurosurgery & Psychiatry. 2008;79: 368-376.

22) C: Pill-rolling tremor of 5-10 Hz

The resting pill-rolling (supination-pronation) tremor of Parkinson's disease is 4-6 Hz, whereas essential tremor is characteristically 5-10 Hz. Camptocormia describes a flexed posture that appears on standing or walking, but can be corrected by lying down supine, and is seen in Parkinson's disease.

Jankovic J. Parkinson's disease: clinical features and diagnosis.Journal of Neurology, Neurosurgery and Psychiatry. 2008;79:368-376

23) B. COMT inhibitor

The management of Parkinson's Disease (PD), as with many conditions in medicine, invariably requires a multi-disciplinary approach (examiners love this term in OSCEs!), although pharmacological treatment plays a key role. Such drug treatments include dopamine receptor agonists and levodopa. Levodopa is commenced only when symptoms become distressing for the patient and are severe enough to significantly impact on the patient's quality of life. The delayed use of this drug is mainly because of its end-of-dose deterioration effects, whereby its efficacy reduces the longer it has been used. In order to minimise the dose of levodopa given to PD patients, and reduce the risk of associated side-effects, it is often prescribed in conjunction with DOPA decarboxylase inhibitors (e.g. carbidopa), COMT inhibitors (entacapone and tolcapone) or MAO-B inhibitors (rasagiline and selegiline).

24) E: Shy-Drager syndrome

Parkinsonism with early manifestations of autonomic dysfunction suggests a diagnosis of multi-system atrophy (also known as Shy-Drager syndrome). This patient's wife left him recently because of sexual dysfunction. Measurements of standing and lying blood pressure highlight the presence of postural hypotension as the drop in systolic blood pressure is more than 20 mmHg.

Jankovic J. Parkinson's disease: clinical features and diagnosis.Journal of Neurology, Neurosurgery and Psychiatry. 2008;79:368-376

25) A: Lamotrigine

This is a typical case of tonic-clonic seizures. Recall that epilepsy is defined as a history of 2 or more unprovoked seizures (any healthy person without epilepsy can have a seizure provoked by severe hypoxia, hyperthermia, electrolyte imbalances, drugs etc). Seizures can be classified as simple or complex and partial or generalised. Complex seizures are associated with a loss or disturbance of consciousness, whilst simple seizures are not. Partial seizures involve a focal area of brain, whilst generalised seizures involve the entire brain (both hemispheres). Partial seizures can become *secondarily generalised* when the initial focus of hyperexcitability spreads across the rest of the brain. Thus, a tonic-clonic seizure, which is a form of complex, generalized seizure, can be primary or secondary.

During the initial tonic phase, muscles turn rigid, including those of the larynx, causing the individual to collapse with a yelp as they lose consciousness. The clonic phase ensues, and accounts for the limbs shaking, during which the individual may experience urinary and/or faecal incontinence and lateral tongue biting. During the post-ictal phase, the individual feels confused and tired for at least several hours, has muscle aches and importantly cannot recall what happened during the seizure.

Both sodium valproate and lamotrigine are appropriate first line therapies for tonic-clonic seizures. However, due to the teratogenic effect of sodium valproate (increased risk of neural tube defects in the developing fetus), this drug should be avoided in all women of child-bearing age. Topiramate and carbamazepine are appropriate second-line agents, whilst ethosuximide is utilised in absence seizures.

26) B: Absence epilepsy

The scenario is typical of absence epilepsy, which represents recurrent primary generalised non-convulsive seizures occurring up to 200 times/day. The ictal EEG manifestation characteristic of absence seizure is the 2.5-4 Hz bilateral spike and slow-wave synchronous discharge, which usually lasts for around 10 seconds (range of 4-20 seconds). The pathophysiological mechanisms underpinning absence seizures are thought to be aberrant electrical activity of hyper-excitable cortico-thalamocortical loops.

Crunelli V and Leresche N. Childhood absence epilepsy: genes, channels, neurons and networks. Nature Reviews Neuroscience. 2002;3:371-382

27) C: Absence seizures occur in around 5% of patients with JME

Juvenile Myoclonic Epilepsy (JME) is an idiopathic, generalised epilepsy encompassing myoclonic jerks (100%), generalised tonic-clonic seizures (90-95%) and less commonly absence seizures (in 40% of cases). It is hereditary with a positive family history in up to 50% of patients.

Myoclonic jerks are brief muscle contractions, usually affecting the shoulders and arms. The jerks can be singular or repetitive and are often worse in the morning – patients may complain of inadvertently flinging their cereal bowl (hence the branded name 'Kellogg's epilepsy').

Renganathan R and Delanty N. Juvenile myoclonic epilepsy: under-appreciated and under-diagnosed. Postgraduate Medical Journal. 2003; 79:78-80

28) E: 10 years

Temporal lobe epilepsy consists of recurrent complex, partial seizures arising in the temporal lobes of the brain. In approximately 80% of cases, the seizures are preceded by auras, which consist of illusions (distortions of incoming sensory data) or hallucinations (the internal generation of sensory perceptions independent of incoming stimuli) that can span multiple different sensory modalities. Auras may be olfactory, gustatory, visual, auditory, somatosensory, autonomic or psychic symptoms. Examples of psychic auras include déjà vu or jamais vu, the strange sense of familiarity or unfamiliarity, respectively.

These auras are in fact simple partial seizures as their aetiology is thought to be aberrant electrical activity affecting focal areas of cerebral cortex arising in the context of intact consciousness. As the electrical activity spreads, the patient loses awareness of his or her surroundings, so the partial seizure becomes complex. Patients typically stare ahead blankly and display stereotyped behavioural patterns called automatisms, such as lip smacking, chewing, swallowing and fumbling with their clothing. After a few minutes, the patient regains consciousness, appears disoriented and has no memory of what happened, though any preceding auras can usually be recalled.

All drivers newly diagnosed with epilepsy have a responsibility to inform the DVLA. Group 1 drivers (ordinary motor vehicles) with epileptic attacks whilst awake must remain seizure free for at least 1 year (with or without anticonvulsants) before they can reapply for their driver's license. Patients with seizures whilst asleep may also reapply for a group 1 license after at least 1 year. However, providing that no seizures have occurred whilst awake for at least 3 years since the original attack, such patients may still apply for their license even though seizures whilst asleep continue to occur. Group 2 drivers (heavy goods vehicles) must remain free from any kind of seizure (awake or asleep) *with no anticonvulsants* for at least 10 years before they can reapply for their HGV license.

Drivers Medical Group, DVLA. For Medical Practitioners: At a glance Guide to the current Medical Standards of Fitness to Drive. 2011.

29) E: Is associated with thymoma in 60% of cases

The patient has myasthenia gravis (MG), which is an autoimmune condition characterised by a disruption in neuromuscular transmission secondary to depletion of nicotinic acetylcholine receptors (nAChR) on the post-synaptic membranes. About 85% of cases are associated with anti-nAChR antibodies, whilst 5-8% of patients have antibodies targeting muscle specific tyrosine kinase. The hallmark of MG is muscle fatigability whereby repeated muscular contractions exacerbate muscle weakness. This is in contrast to Lambert-Eaton myasthenic syndrome, a paraneoplastic phenomenon in about half of cases (usually associated with small cell lung cancer), where muscular strength improves following repetitive muscle contractions. When the age of onset of MG is below 40-50 years, women are more commonly affected, but the reverse is true in late onset MG.

The Tensilon test is a useful investigation for MG, and involves the intravenous injection of the short-acting anticholinesterase, edrophonium chloride. Edrophonium transiently improves MG symptoms by inhibiting cholinesterase enzymes, which raises the concentration of acetylcholine and improves signal transmission within the neuromuscular junctions. As MG can be associated with thymoma (in 10-15% not 60% of patients), a CT chest is recommended in all patients.

Jacob S, Viegas S, Lashley D and Hilton-Jones D. The Bare essentials: Myasthenia gravis and other neuromuscular junction disorders. Pract Neurol. 2009:9;364-371.

30) B: Syringomyelia

In syringomyelia, a tubular enlargement of the central canal of the spinal cord, called a syrinx, develops. The syrinx can form anywhere in the cord or even the brainstem (in which case it would be called syringobulbia), but in this clinical scenario is localised to the cervical cord. Since decussating spinothalamic nerves form part of the thin anterior commissure of the cord, lying in close proximity to the central canal, these are amongst the first fibres to be damaged by the growing syrinx.

This accounts for the selectively diminished pain and temperature sensation bilaterally, which is unlikely to be noticed by the patient as fine tactile sensation is still preserved because the dorsal columns are often spared. As the syrinx continues to expand, the adjacent ventral horns become damaged, leading to lower motor neuron signs at the same level. This explains the hand signs.

Nolte J. The Human Brain: An Introduction to Its Functional Anatomy, Fifth Edition. Mosby. 2002.

31) A: High-dose corticosteroids

The patient has pituitary apoplexy, which is characterized by haemorrhagic necrosis or infarction of a pre-existing pituitary adenoma. This creates a mass effect, which results in compression of adjacent structures within the cavernous sinus, such as the oculomotor nerve, which is commonly involved (cranial nerves IV and VI compression is less common in pituitary apoplexy).

Patients may also present with visual field defects, which can be due to any of optic chiasm, tract or nerve compression resulting in bitemporal, contralateral homonymous hemianopia or monocular visual field defects, respectively.

Left untreated, patients can deteriorate rapidly, one reason being cardiovascular collapse due to secondary adrenocortical insufficiency (as there is a hypopituitarism, which causes ACTH levels to plummet). This necessitates the prompt administration of high dose intravenous hydrocortisone.

Although patients with pituitary apoplexy may require mannitol to manage intracranial hypertension, this comes secondary to steroid replacement. Vasopressors and inotropic support is considered when the patient has already deteriorated significantly due to cardiovascular instability despite use of steroids.

Oral nimodipine is employed in subarachnoid haemorrhage (SAH), which can indeed mimic pituitary apoplexy (thunderclap doesn't always equal SAH), in order to counteract vasospasm and cerebral ischaemia. Interestingly, patients with pituitary apoplexy can develop subarachnoid haemorrhage as blood within the pituitary adenoma ruptures through a defect in the encasing tumour capsule, leaking into the subarachnoid space.

Rajasekarant S, Vanderpump M, Baldeweg S, Drake W, Reddy N, Lanyon M, et al. UK guidelines for the management of pituitary apoplexy: pituitary apoplexy guidelines development group. Clin Endocrinol (Oxf) 2011;74:9-20

Kerr JM and Wierman ME. Pituitary apoplexy: New guidelines refine best practise, but some areas remain uncertain. British Medical Journal. 2011;342:668-669.

Wohaibi M AL, Russell NA and Ferayan A AL. Pituitary apoplexy presenting as massive subarachnoid haemorrhage. Journal of Neurology, Neurosurgery and Psychiatry. 2000;69:700-701.

32) D: 9

The patient's GCS is 9/15 (E2V2M5)

Glasgow coma scale

Eye opening:

Spontaneous	4
To speech	3
To pain	2
None	1

Best Verbal Response:

Orientated	5
Confused	4
Inappropriate	3
Incomprehensible	2
None	1

Best Motor Response:

Obeying commands	6
Localising	5
Withdrawing	4
Flexing	3
Extending	2
None	1

Teasdale G and Jennett B. Assessment of coma and impaired consciousness. The Lancet. 1974;2:81-84.

33) A: Lateral cutaneous nerve of the thigh

Meralgia paraesthetica is a nerve entrapment syndrome due to compression of the lateral cutaneous nerve of the thigh as it passes through the inguinal ligament. Patients often complain of a burning pain affecting the anterolateral part of the thigh.

34) C: Adductor pollicis

The median nerve innervates the LOAF muscles of the hand (lateral two lumbricals, opponens pollicis, abductor pollicis brevis and flexor pollicis brevis), whereas adductor pollicis is innervated by the ulnar nerve.

35) B: Contralateral homonymous superior quadrantanopia

Each optic tract carries nerve fibres from the ipsilateral temporal retina and contralateral nasal retina, which collaboratively represent the contralateral half of the visual field. Thus, an optic tract lesion would produce a contralateral homonymous hemianopia.

The neurons of each optic tract terminate in the ipsilateral lateral geniculate nucleus (LGN) of the thalamus. During their path to the visual cortex, the LGN nerve fibres fan out to form the optic radiation. The inferior part of the optic radiation forms Meyer's loop, which is comprised of fibres that move antero-laterally towards the temporal pole before sharply curving posteriorly towards the occipital lobes. Damage to Meyer's loop owing to a temporal lobe lesion would produce a contralateral homonymous superior quadrantanopia. A contralateral homonymous inferior quadrantanopia would be produced following damage to the superior components of the optic radiation, which cross the parietal lobes. Damage to the occipital lobes would produce loss of the contralateral half of the visual field with macular sparing.

Nolte J. The Human Brain: An Introduction to Its Functional Anatomy, Fifth Edition. Mosby. 2002.

36) E: The most common variant of MND is primary lateral sclerosis

Motor neurone disease (MND) is characterised by progressive destruction of motor neurones and invariably carries a poor prognosis with an average predicted survival of 2-4 years from the onset of symptoms.

The most common variant is amyotrophic lateral sclerosis (ALS) which involves degeneration of both upper and lower motor neurones. When only the upper motor neurones are destroyed, the variant is primary lateral sclerosis, whereas when only the lower motor neurones are destroyed, the variant is progressive muscular atrophy.

The most common clinical presentation of MND is that of progressive wasting and weakness of the muscles of the limbs. If the lower limbs are involved, patients may complain of stumbling or tripping over frequently, or with difficulty climbing stairs. If the upper limbs are involved, problems with opening bottles, buttoning up a shirt and writing can be affected. In around 20% of patients, bulbar onset is seen, first manifesting as slurring of speech, followed by difficulty in swallowing, especially liquids (neurological causes of dysphagia makes swallowing liquids harder than solids, whilst the reverse is true for mechanical causes).

Clinical findings that should raise suspicion of MND are the existence of hyper-reflexia in a wasted limb (as in ALS), along with the absence of sensory signs, and particularly if there is relentless progression of the patient's condition. Note, however, a combination of upper and lower motor neurone signs may also be seen in spinal radiculomyelopathies where there is compression of both cord and spinal roots.

McDermott CJ and Shaw PJ. Diagnosis and management of motor neurone disease. British Medical Journal. 2008;336:658-662.

Longmore M, Wilkinson IB, Davidson EH, Foulkes A and Mafi AR. Oxford Handbook of Clinical Medicine. Eighth edition. Oxford.2010.

37) E: Platelet count of 110 x 10⁹/litre

The patient's symptoms suggest meningitis (it is not possible to differentiate between a viral or bacterial cause on the basis of the patient's initial symptoms, although bacterial meningitis is often more severe). A platelet count of less than 50 is a contraindication to lumbar puncture due to the risk of an epidural haematoma. The first 4 options are signs suggestive of raised intracranial pressure (ICP). Proceeding with a lumbar puncture if the raised ICP is secondary to a space occupying lesion would result in coning (i.e. herniation of the cerebellar tonsils across the foramen magnum), progressing to brainstem compression and death.

National Institute for Health and Clinical Excellence. 2010. Bacterial meningitis and meningococcal septicaemia. CG102. London: National Institute for Health and Clinical Excellence.

38) B: Herpes simplex encephalitis

Herpes simplex encephalitis (HSE) is a rare condition but carries a very high mortality. 90% of cases of HSE in children and adults are due to HSV-1, which characteristically affects the temporal lobes, often asymmetrically. As well as standard resuscitative measures, specific management of HSE requires 10mg/kg acyclovir three times daily for 14 days, given intravenously. Such treatment can lower the mortality from 70% to around 20-30%.

Kennedy PGE and Chaudhuri A. Herpes simplex encephalitis. Journal of Neurology, Neurosurgery and Psychiatry. 2002;73:237-238.

39) A: Radial nerve – spiral groove

The radial nerve is a continuation of the posterior cord of the brachial plexus, which arises from a combination of C5-T1 nerve roots. In the axilla, it sends a motor branch to the triceps and sensory branches to the skin overlying triceps and posterior forearm.

It subsequently runs along the spiral groove of the humerus, whereby it emerges adjacent to the lateral epicondyle and sends motor innervation to the brachioradialis muscle. It then divides to form the posterior interosseous nerve, which innervates the supinator and continues distally to supply the wrist and finger extensors, and sensory branches, which travels down the forearm to become superficial at the wrist, and supplies skin overlying the first dorsal interosseous.

A lesion at various points along the course of the radial nerve would therefore be expected to give rise to varying patterns of motor and sensory disturbance.

40) A: Ramsay-Hunt syndrome

Ramsay-Hunt syndrome is due to the reactivation of varicella zoster virus in the distribution of the facial nerve. The rash on the ear is due to the fact that the facial nerve provides sensory innervation to a small patch of skin in this region, although a rash may also be seen on the tongue or soft palate.

Asking patients with facial nerve palsies to raise their eyebrows will enable one to differentiate an upper from a lower motor neurone lesion. If a patient retains the ability to raise the eyebrow and wrinkle the forehead on the affected side, then the facial palsy is due to an upper motor neurone lesion. The reason for this is because the facial nucleus, located in the caudal pons, *representing the upper part of the face* is supplied by upper motor neurones arising from the right and left motor cortex. Therefore, even if upper motor neurones on one side become damaged, that part of the facial nucleus responsible for raising the eyebrows still remains innervated by a set of upper motor cortical neurones on the unaffected side.

On the other hand, failure to raise the eyebrow and wrinkle the forehead in the context of a facial palsy signifies a lower motor neurone facial nerve lesion.

Sweeney CJ and Gilden DH. Ramsay Hunt syndrome. Journal of Neurology, Neurosurgery and Psychiatry. 2001;71:149-154.

Gastroenterology Questions

1) A 34-year old male presents with a 3-month history of bloody diarrhoea and weight loss. He subsequently undergoes a flexible sigmoidoscopy, which reveals uniform inflammatory changes extending proximally from the rectal mucosa towards the sigmoid colon. The endoscopist takes multiple biopsies of the inflamed mucosa.

Which of the following histological features would not be expected?

A. Crypt abscesses
B. Goblet cell depletion
C. Superficial mucosal inflammation
D. Granuloma formation
E. Basal plasmacytosis

2) A 66-year old lady presents with lethargy, painless jaundice and pruritus.

On examination, there is xanthelasma and yellowing of the sclera. Investigations reveal:

Hb	11.6	(11.6-14g/dl)
MCV	86	(80-100fl)
Platelets	250	(150-400x 10^9/L)
WBC	7.3	(4-12x 10^9/L)
ALT	86	(5-40 IU/L)
Bilirubin	82	(3-17 micromol/l)
ALP	430	(30-120 IU/L)
CA19-9	Normal	

Which of the following antibodies is most strongly associated with this condition?

A. Anti-nuclear antibodies
B. Anti-mitochondrial antibodies
C. Anti-smooth muscle antibodies
D. Anti-Ro antibodies
E. Anti-La antibodies

3) A 28-year old Caucasian male presents with a 4-month history of intermittent episodes of diarrhoea, intermittent cramping abdominal pain and 8 kg weight loss.

He undergoes a colonoscopy, which shows a cobblestone appearance to the large bowel.

What is the most likely diagnosis?

A. Ischaemic Colitis
B. Coeliac disease
C. Pseudomembranous colitis
D. Ulcerative colitis
E. Crohn's disease

4) A 38-year old male with newly diagnosed Crohn's disease is commenced on azathioprine for maintenance of remission.

Six weeks into treatment, he develops a sore throat, cough, lethargy and easy bruising.

Bloods, which were completely normal prior to treatment, now reveal:

Hb	9.5 g/dl
White cell count	1.2 x 10^9/L
Platelets	60 x 10^9/L

Deficiency in which of the following enzymes is most likely to have caused this clinical picture?

A. Xanthine oxidase
B. Thiopurine methyltransferase
C. Glucose 6-phosphate dehydrogenase
D. Dihydrofolate reductase
E. Hypoxanthine-guanine phosphoribosyl-transferase

5) Which of the following is the most common extra-intestinal manifestation of inflammatory bowel disease?

A. Enteropathic arthritis
B. Erythema nodosum
C. Pyoderma gangrenosum
D. Anterior uveitis
E. Nephrolithiasis

6) A 48-year old gentleman presents with fatigue, pruritus and right upper quadrant discomfort.

Past medical history includes ulcerative colitis. Investigations reveal:

Hb	12.0 g/dl	(11.6-14g/dl)
MCV	84 fl	(80-100fl)
Platelets	350 x 10⁹/L	(150-400x 10⁹/L)
WBC	8.2 x 10⁹/L	(4-12x 10⁹/L)
ALT	92	(5-40 IU/L)
Bilirubin	67	(3-17 micromol/l)
ALP	730	(30-120 IU/L)
Gamma GT	530	(10-45 IU/L)

ERCP – Multiple intra- and extra-hepatic strictures and beading of the biliary ducts

What is the most likely diagnosis?

A. Primary sclerosing cholangitis
B. Primary biliary cirrhosis
C. Pancreatic cancer
D. Caroli disease
E. Gallstone-related liver disease

7) Which of the following statements regarding ulcerative colitis is FALSE?

A. It has a prevalence of approximately 100-200/100,000
B. It is associated with an increased risk of colon cancer
C. Inflammation is commonly restricted to the mucosa
D. Smoking is associated with a reduced risk of ulcerative colitis
E. Inflammation only affects the rectum and colon

8) A 24-year old male student is referred to the gastroenterology clinic. He presents with a 6-month history of weight loss, bloating, lethargy and bulky stools that is very difficult to flush.

Bloods reveal:

Hb	9.6 g/dl	(11.6-14g/dl)
MCV	108.0	(80-100fl)
Platelets	460 x 10^9/L	(150-400x 10^9/L)
White cell count	8.4 x 10^9/L	(4-12x 10^9/L)
Anti-endomysial Ab	Positive	

Which of the following is the next most appropriate investigation?

A. Colonoscopy and terminal ileum biopsy
B. Abdominal X-ray
C. Small bowel enteroclysis
D. Double-contrast barium enema
E. Oesophago-gastro-duodenoscopy and duodenal biopsy

9) A 58-year old lady presents with a 6-week history of diarrhoea and paroxysmal episodes of facial flushing and wheeze.

On examination, abdomen is soft, non-tender and there is a 2cm irregular hepatomegaly.

Investigations reveal:

24-hour urine 5-hydroxyindoleacetic acid levels: 30 mg (normal: 2-7mg)

Where is the primary tumour most likely to be located?

A. Cecum
B. Appendix
C. Rectum
D. Liver
E. Lung

10) A 38-year old male is brought to the emergency department with sudden onset, severe central chest pain. This was precipitated following repeated bouts of retching and vomiting after binge drinking.

The attending physician performs a clinical examination and notices a 'crackling feeling' as he palpates the patient's chest.

What is the most appropriate diagnostic investigation?

A. Barium swallow
B. Echocardiogram
C. Gastrografin swallow
D. Capsule endoscopy
E. Oesophagogastroduodenoscopy

11) A 67-year old gentleman is brought to see his GP by his concerned wife. She has noticed that he has become progressively confused and lethargic over the last 5-6 months. During that period, he has also experienced relentless diarrhoea and progressive loss of appetite.

On examination, there is a bilaterally symmetrical, well-demarcated erythematous scaly rash on the hands, arms and around the neck. His wife comments that this is new.

He is disorientated to place and time and has an MMSE score of 20/30.

Deficiency in which of the following is most likely to account for this patient's symptoms?

A. Vitamin B1
B. Vitamin B2
C. Vitamin B3
D. Vitamin B6
E. Vitamin B12

12) A 12-year old boy presents to clinic with jaundice. Slit-lamp examination reveals Kayser-Fleischer rings.

What is the most appropriate treatment?

A. Azathioprine
B. Desferrioxamine
C. Prednisolone
D. Penicillamine
E. Methotrexate

13) A 47-year old woman is seen in clinic because of a 1-month history of progressively worsening intermittent epigastric pain. The pain is worst at night, typically waking her up from sleep and is often relieved by food. It is associated with belching, bloating and early satiety.

She undergoes an Oesophago-Gastro-Duodenoscopy, which reveals a peptic ulcer at the duodenal cap. A rapid urease test is positive for *Helicobacter Pylori*.

Which of the following is the most appropriate treatment?

A. Omeprazole, amoxicillin and clarithromycin
B. Omeprazole, metronizadole and clindamycin
C. Vancomycin and omeprazole
D. Lansoprazole, ciprofloxacin and amoxicillin
E. Lansoprazole, ceftriaxone and metronidazole

14) A 38-year old lady presents to the medical assessment unit with a 2-day history of worsening abdominal pain and confusion.

Past medical history includes liver cirrhosis secondary to alcohol excess.

On examination, the abdomen is very distended and shifting dullness test is positive. There is significant tenderness with guarding in the right peri-umbilical region.

Heart rate is 110/min regular, blood pressure is 108/68 mmHg and temperature is 38.3 degrees.

An ascitic tap is performed, which reveals a neutrophil count of 400 cells/microlitre.

Which of the following types of bacteria is most likely to be cultured from the ascitic fluid?

A. Gram-positive facultative aerobic bacilli
B. Gram-negative aerobic cocci
C. Gram-negative anaerobic cocci
D. Gram-negative aerobic bacilli
E. Gram-negative facultative anaerobic bacilli

15) A 45-year old gentleman presents to his GP with a 6-week history of epigastric discomfort, nausea and bloating. His symptoms have failed to settle despite having taken regular gaviscon.

Past medical history is unremarkable.

Assuming that the local prevalence of H. Pylori is 15%, what is the next most appropriate line of management?

A. C-13 urea breath test and H. Pylori eradication, if positive
B. Referral for an urgent oesophago-gastroduodenoscopy (OGD) and rapid urease test
C. Urgent CT-abdomen and pelvis with contrast
D. Trial of proton pump inhibitor for 4 to 8 weeks and review
E. Reassure and recommend other antacid treatment

16) You review a 39-year old patient in A and E who has presented with malaena.

On examination, he is maintaining his own airway, talking in full sentences, appears anxious and is cool and clammy to touch.

Observations are: heart rate 132/min regular, blood pressure is 126/90 mmHg, temperature is 36.8 degrees, oxygen saturation is 96% on air.

Assuming he is 70kg, approximately how much blood has this patient lost?

A. <750ml
B. 750-1500ml
C. 1500-2000ml
D. 2000-2500ml
E. 2500-3000ml

17) You review a 24-year old male student who presented to A and E an hour ago with acute severe, central, colicky abdominal pain.

It started around 3 days ago, but has become progressively worse and more frequent. He has had multiple previous similar episodes over the past few months but these have been self-limiting unlike the one on this occasion. He normally opens his bowels once a day, but hasn't opened his bowels since 4 days ago. He has vomited 5 times over the last 1 day.

On examination, the patient intermittently clutches his abdomen due to pain. The patient is very tender in the periumbilical region with guarding, but the abdomen is otherwise soft. Bowel sounds are hyperactive. There is evidence of pigmentation around the lips and in the buccal mucosa.

What is the most likely underlying diagnosis?

A. Small bowel lymphoma
B. Osler-Weber-Rendu syndrome
C. Lynch syndrome
D. Familial adenomatous polyposis
E. Peutz-Jegher's syndrome

18) You have been called to resus to urgently review a patient who has presented with haematemesis and haematochezia.

After being resuscitated, she is transferred to the endoscopy unit for an urgent Oesophago-Gastro-Duodenoscopy.

Findings at endoscopy reveal an actively bleeding duodenal ulcer, which is treated with multiple local adrenaline injections and thermal coagulation.

What is the next most appropriate line of treatment?

A. Intravenous bolus of omeprazole 80mg followed by an infusion of 8mg/hour
B. Intravenous omeprazole, cefuroxime and metronidazole
C. Give intravenous 2mg bolus of terlipressin, followed by an infusion of 2mg/4hourly
D. Observe and perform planned re-endoscopy after 24 hours
E. Observe and repeat endoscopy only if patient rebleeds

19) A 54-year old male patient is reviewed in clinic. He was recently diagnosed with liver cirrhosis secondary to excess alcohol intake and a screening OGD has confirmed the presence of multiple medium-sized oesophageal varices.

There has been no recent history of haematemesis.

Which of the following is the most appropriate treatment for primary prophylaxis of variceal haemorrhage?

A. Terlipressin
B. Bisoprolol
C. Spironolactone
D. Propanolol
E. Vasopressin

20) Which of the following cells produce somatostatin?

A. Alpha cells
B. Beta cells
C. Delta cells
D. Parietal cells
E. G cells

21) A 68-year old gentleman presents to his GP with painless jaundice and unintentional weight loss.

He has noticed that his stools have become pale and his urine dark.

Which one of the following tumour markers is most likely to be grossly elevated?

A. AFP
B. CEA
C. hCG
D. CA 125
E. CA 19-9

22) A 40-year old gentleman presents with a 4-month history of diarrhoea, weight loss, polyarthalgia and colicky abdominal pain.

On examination, there is evidence of occulomasticatory myorrhythmia.

OGD and jejunal biopsies show a lamina propria infiltrated with PAS-positive macrophages.

What is the most likely diagnosis?

A. Whipple's disease
B. Tropical sprue
C. Bacterial overgrowth syndrome
D. Coeliac disease
E. Autoimmune enteropathy

23) A 68-year old arteriopath is admitted to hospital with acute severe abdominal pain.

A diagnosis of ischaemic colitis is suspected.

Which of the following radiological signs would be most supportive of this diagnosis?

A. Sentinel loop sign
B. String sign of Kantor
C. Thumbprinting
D. Transverse colon diameter of 10cm
E. Corkscrew sign

24) You are presented with the following liver function tests in someone who has presented with evidence of decompensated liver disease:

AST   250   (6-40IU/L)
ALT   120   (6-40IU/L)
Bilirubin 48   (3-20 micromol/L)
ALP   240   (30-120IU/L)

Which of the following is the most likely aetiology?

A. Gallstones
B. Alcohol excess
C. Paracetamol overdose
D. Viral Hepatitis
E. Wilson's disease

25) A 76-year old gentleman presents to the emergency department with a 24-hour history of sudden onset severe central abdominal pain. He also reports a 6-month history of PR bleeding and intermittent, transient abdominal pain precipitated by eating.

He is a heavy smoker with a past medical history that includes ischaemic heart disease and peripheral vascular disease. He drinks around 26 units alcohol/week. On examination, he looks very unwell with evidence of generalised peritonitis. Blood tests reveal:

Hb 10.4 (12-16g/dl)	Na⁺ 136 (135-145mmol/l)
MCV 74 (80-100)	K⁺ 4.8 (3.5-5mmol/l)
Platelets 260 (150-400x 10⁹/L)	Urea 8.2 (2.2-8.3mmol/l)
Lactate 9.0 (0.5-1.6mmol/l)	Creatinine 96 (60-100micromol/l)
Amylase 120 (<100U/L)	

What is the most likely diagnosis?

A. Perforated duodenal ulcer
B. Toxic megacolon
C. Acute cholecystitis
D. Acute pancreatitis
E. Acute mesenteric ischaemia

26) A 22-year old female student presents to the assessment unit with haematemesis. On further questioning, she reports she had been vomiting and retching repeatedly following a binge drink, before she noticed streaks of blood in her vomit.

She has recently been started on diclofenac for tennis elbow by her GP.

On examination, she is alert and orientated, heart rate is 68/min, blood pressure is 126/80 mmHg, oxygen saturations 98% on air and temperature is 36.9 degrees.

What is the most likely diagnosis?

A. Gastric ulcer
B. Duodenal ulcer
C. Boerhaaves syndrome
D. Oesophageal varices
E. Mallory-Weiss tear

27) A 43-year old lady presents to clinic with a 3-month history of dysphagia to solid foods, which has more recently progressed to liquids. She has also been complaining of heartburn and intermittent central chest pain.

The gastroenterologist orders a barium swallow, which the radiologist reports as having a "birds-beak appearance".

What is the most likely diagnosis?

A. Oesophageal cancer
B. Barrett's oesophagus
C. Achalasia
D. Nutcracker oesophagus
E. Gastro-oesophageal reflux disease

28) A 32-year old female is admitted under the medical take with a 3-week history of diarrhoea and generalised, colicky abdominal pains.

She has recently returned from a holiday in the United States, which included a trek in the Rocky Mountains.

Stool is positive for Giardia cysts.

What is the most appropriate treatment?

A. Ciprofloxacin
B. Vancomycin
C. Fluconazole
D. Metronidazole
E. Streptomycin

29) A patient has recently been diagnosed with coeliac disease.

Which HLA haplotype is most strongly associated with this condition?

A. DR3
B) DR4
C) DQ2
D) DQ8
E) B27

30) A 65-year old man with a past medical history of Hypertension, Type 2 Diabetes Mellitus and Atrial Fibrillation presents to clinic with a 6-month history of bloating, lethargy and 5kg unintentional weight loss.

In the past week, he has noticed 2 episodes of fresh blood passed with defaecation and has generally noticed passage of looser motions.

He is an ex-smoker; his current medications include: Amlodipine, Digoxin, Metformin, Lansoprazole and Warfarin.

Clinical examination, including rectal examination, is unremarkable.

His blood tests are as follows:

INR	3.1	
Hb	10.3g/dl	(13.5-18.0g/dl)
MCV	82.1fl	(80-102fl)
Platelets	512 x10^9/l	(140-450 x10^9/l)
CRP	31	(<10)

What is the most likely diagnosis?

A. Acute Diverticulitis
B. Diverticular Colitis
C. Ischaemic Colitis
D. Clostridium Difficile Infection
E. Rectal Carcinoma

31) An 80-year old nursing home resident with a known diagnosis of vascular dementia and severe rheumatoid arthritis is noted by the nursing staff to have fresh blood and clots mixed with her stool.

She has previously documented endoscopic evidence of diverticulae 10 years ago, but denies any symptoms of abdominal pain or pyrexia.

Which investigation should be performed?

A. Mesenteric Angiography
B. Colonoscopy
C. Capsule Endoscopy
D. CT scan
E. CEA blood test

32) Which of the following is true regarding diverticular disease:

A. Caffeine is a risk factor for the development of colonic diverticulae.
B. Iron deficiency anaemia can be caused by uncomplicated diverticulosis.
C. Surgical resection is curative for diverticular colitis
D. Diverticulosis is the commonest cause of massive haematochezia
E. The presence of a meckels diverticulum is associated with the development of diverticulae in older life

33) Which of the following statements is true regarding the pathophysiology and treatment of complications associated with diverticulosis?

A. Obesity is a risk factor for diverticular bleeding
B. Additional symptoms of lethargy are more indicative of complicated diverticulitis
C. The risk of perforation in complicated diverticulitis is more common in left sided diverticular disease than right sided
D. Diverticular colitis can be managed with steroids
E. Diverticulosis is a risk factor for the development of adenomatous polyps.

34) Which of the following statements regarding paracetamol overdose is incorrect?

A. The earliest time a reliable plasma paracetamol level can be measured is 8 hours after the time of overdose
B. Hepatocellular damage is maximal 3-4 days post-overdose
C. N-acetylcysteine should be commenced immediately in patients presenting 8-36 hours after an overdose even if a paracetamol level is not yet available
D. Activated charcoal is only effective if given within 1 hour of overdose
E. Patients taking liver enzyme inducing drugs are at high risk of hepatic damage

35) A 21-year old male student sees his GP because he has noticed that he has turned yellow in colour.

He reports that this has happened on multiple occasions in the past.

He is recovering from an upper respiratory tract infection at present and is otherwise well.

Investigations reveal:

Hb	13.0 g/dl	(13.5-18.0g/dl)
MCV	88 fl	(80-102fl)
Platelets	310 x 10^9/L	(140-450 x10^9/l)
WBC	10.2 x 10^9/L	(4-12x 10^9/L)

ALT	38	(5-40 IU/L)
Bilirubin	64	(3-17 micromol/l)
ALP	60	(30-120 IU/L)

Direct Coombs test: negative
Blood film: normal

Unconjugated bilirubin: Elevated
Conjugated bilirubin: Normal

What is the most likely diagnosis?

A. Dubin-Johnson syndrome
B. Gilbert's syndrome
C. Criggler-Najar syndrome
D. Hereditary spherocytosis
E. G6PD-deficiency

36) An 83-year old lady is treated in hospital for a severe community-acquired pneumonia with intravenous antibiotics.

One week into her hospital stay, she develops diarrhoea and diffuse abdominal pains. *Clostridium Difficile* toxin is detected in her stool sample.

What is the most appropriate treatment?

A. Intravenous vancomycin for 10 days
B. Oral ciprofloxacin for 7 days
C. Oral metronidazole for 4 days
D. Oral metronidazole for 10 days
E. Intravenous co-amoxiclav for 10 days

37) A 62-year old gentleman presents to his GP with a 1-month history of acid reflux. His medication list is as follows:

Amlodipine 10mg once daily
Isosorbide mononitrate 10mg twice daily

Oxybutynin 5 mg twice daily
Amitriptylline 25 mg once at night
Digoxin 125 micrograms once daily

Stopping which of the above drugs is least likely to have a beneficial effect on this patient's heartburn?

A. Amlodipine
B. Isosorbide mononitrate
C. Oxybutynin
D. Amitriptylline
E. Digoxin

38) A 43-year old patient presents with a 3-month history of lethargy and joint pains. Past medical history includes diabetes mellitus controlled with insulin.

On examination, the patient is tanned, has evidence of palmar erythema, multiple spider naevi on the trunk and yellowing of the sclera.

Investigations reveal:

Hb	11.5 g/dl
MCV	90 fl
Platelets	320 x 10^9/L
Ferritin	1200 microgram/L
Transferrin saturation	52%
Bilirubin	86 micromol/l
ALT	260 IU/L
ALP	430 IU/L

Which chromosome is the genetic abnormality most likely to be located given the above clinical findings?

A. 2
B. 4
C. X
D. 6
E. 8

39) Which of the following statements regarding gastro-oesophageal reflux disease (GORD) is incorrect?

A. Symptoms are typically worse upon lying down, stooping and straining
B. Prolonged GORD increases the risk of oesophageal malignancy
C. Patients should refrain from consuming citrus fruits and tomatoes as these can worse symptoms
D. 24-hour oesophageal pH monitoring represents the gold standard investigation for diagnosing GORD
E. A normal endoscopy excludes a diagnosis of GORD

40) A 76-year old man had symptoms of abdominal pain, constipation and bloating. Although initially presumed to have Irritable Bowel Syndrome, he underwent a colonoscopy revealing extensive sigmoid diverticulosis.

Over the subsequent 2 years, he is complicated by multiple episodes of diverticulitis.

He is admitted with symptoms of pneumaturia and diagnosed with a pelvic diverticular abscess and colo-ureteric fistula.

Which of the following statements regarding treatment is false:

A. Medical management with antibiotics and a high fibre diet is unlikely to achieve a complete resolution of his symptoms.
B. Laparoscopic resection with end-end anastomosis is always the preferred management strategy
C. Whilst mesocolic abscesses can sometimes be managed conservatively without percutaneous drainage, pelvic abscesses nearly always require drainage.
D. Where possible, surgery for acute diverticulitis should be delayed until after recovery from the acute illness.
E. Regarding the use of surgery as a therapeutic option, there is little evidence to suggest a different approach be considered for younger patients with complicated diverticular disease.

Gastroenterology Answers

1) D: Granuloma formation

The most likely diagnosis is ulcerative colitis (UC); a chronic inflammatory condition of the large bowel characterised by relapses and remissions throughout life. Classically, UC first affects the rectum and spreads proximally: 50% of cases are restricted to the rectum, 30% spread towards the splenic flexure and 20% affect the entire large bowel. Although UC is mostly restricted to the large bowel, in cases of an incompetent ileocaecal valve, a backwash ileitis can occur where the terminal ileum becomes involved in the inflammatory process. Unlike UC, Crohns disease:

a) Can affect the gastrointestinal tract anywhere from the mouth to the anus, although it is largely limited to the large bowel and ileum.
b) Typically causes patchy inflammation, with granuloma formation and transmural involvement (in UC, inflammation is usually uniform and superficial)
c) More often causes stricture formation, which is more likely to lead to bowel obstruction (as opposed to perforation which is a commoner complication in UC) and less often causes a bloody diarrhoea
d) Is more frequent in smokers and smoking is associated with relapses. UC, however, is less frequent in smokers and smoking is usually associated with remission.

Collagen deposition is a feature of microscopic colitis, which is typically associated with watery diarrhoea and normal macroscopic features on colonoscopy.

Melanosis Coli is associated with laxative abuse.

Appleman HD. What Are the Critical Histologic Features in the Diagnosis of Ulcerative Colitis? Inflammatory Bowel Disease. 2008; 14:S164-S165

Langan RC, Gotsch PB, Krafczyk MA and Skillinge DD. Ulcerative Colitis: Diagnosis and Treatment. American Family Physician. 2007;76: 1323-30.

Mowat C, Cole A, Windsor A et al. Guidelines for the management of inflammatory bowel disease in adults. Gut. 2011; 60: 571-607

2) B: Anti-mitochondrial antibodies

With the development of obstructive, painless jaundice in an elderly patient with xanthelasma, a diagnosis of primary biliary cirrhosis (PBC) should be amongst the list of differential diagnoses. Pancreatic cancer is unlikely given the normal levels of CA 19-9 tumour marker. PBC is an autoimmune process strongly associated with anti-mitochondrial antibodies.

Lindor KD, Gershwin ME, Poupon R et al. Primary biliary Cirrhosis. Hepatology. 2009;50: 291-308

3) E: Crohn's disease

Although irritable bowel syndrome (IBS) can produce similar symptoms, significant weight loss and abnormal findings on colonoscopy excludes the diagnosis. The classical cobblestone appearance is a consequence of patchy ulceration of large bowel mucosa separating areas of oedema and makes a diagnosis of Crohn's more likely than ulcerative colitis.

Abraham C and Cho JH. Inflammatory Bowel Disease. The New England Journal of Medicine. 2009;361: 2066-78

4) B: Thiopurine methyltransferase

This patient has presented with pancytopenia secondary to azathioprine toxicity. Azathioprine is initially broken down into its active metabolite, 6-mercaptopurine (6-MP), which is subsequently metabolised further by thiopurine methyltransferase (TPMT), xanthine oxidase or hypoxanthine-guanine phosphoribosyl-transferase in three separate biochemical pathways. Although deficiency of any of these three enzymes can lead to azathioprine toxicity, TPMT deficiency is by far the commonest with 1 in 300 people having absent or significantly low TPMT activity. Allopurinol should be stopped in any patient commencing azathioprine as it inhibits xanthine oxidase and accentuates toxic side effects.

Other recognised adverse effects of azathioprine include hypersensitivity reactions (e.g. fever, myalgia, rash), hepatotoxicity, pneumonitis and pancreatitis.

Anstey A, Lennard L, Mayou SC and Kirby JD. Pancytopenia related to azathioprine – an enzyme deficiency caused by a common genetic polymorphism: a review. Journal of the Royal Society of Medicine. 1992;85: 752-6

5) A: Enteropathic arthritis

Inflammatory arthritis is the most common extra-intestinal manifestation of inflammatory bowel disease, with a prevalence ranging from 7 to 25%.

Danese S, Semeraro S, Papa A et al. Extraintestinal manifestations in inflammatory bowel disease. World Journal of Gastroenterology. 2005;11: 7227-36

6) A: Primary sclerosing cholangitis

Primary biliary cirrhosis (PBC) can present very similarly to primary sclerosing cholangitis (PSC), but the combination of the past medical history of ulcerative colitis and the ERCP findings points us towards PSC as the most likely diagnosis. Although only 5% of patients with inflammatory bowel disease have PSC, nearly 80-90% of those with PSC have inflammatory bowel disease. PSC is more strongly associated with ulcerative colitis than Crohn's disease.

Chapman R, Fevery J, Kalloo A et al. Diagnosis and Management of Primary Sclerosing Cholangitis. Hepatology. 2010;51: 660-78

Collins P and Rhodes J. Ulcerative colitis: diagnosis and management. British Medical Journal. 2006;333: 340-43

7) **E: Inflammation only affects the rectum and colon**

Inflammation in UC is not restricted to the large bowel but can affect the terminal ileum. This is referred to as a backwash ileitis and occurs secondary to incompetence of the ileocaecal valve. Patients with ulcerative colitis are at increased risk of colorectal cancer, and this risk increases with the duration of the disease process. Consequently, certain UC patients are recommended to have surveillance colonoscopies in order to identify the development of potentially malignant colorectal lesions.

Danese S and Fiocchi C. Ulcerative Colitis. The New England Journal of Medicine. 2011;356: 1713-25.

8) **E: Oesophago-gastro-duodenoscopy and duodenal biopsy**

This patient presents with symptoms of malabsorption, of which coeliac disease is the most common cause in the UK.

Coeliac disease is an autoimmune, T-cell mediated, gluten-sensitive enteropathy predominantly affecting the duodenum and jejunum. This patient has a macrocytic anaemia caused by reduced folate absorption (which normally occurs mainly in the jejunum) and has steatorrhoea secondary to fat malabsorption. Patients with coeliac disease are typically positive for anti-endomysial and anti-TTG antibodies. However, as these auto-antibodies are IgA immunoglobulins, false negative results can potentially arise in patients with IgA deficiency, explaining why total IgA levels should always be measured.

The next most appropriate investigation is OGD and duodenal biopsy, which represents the gold-standard investigation for coeliac disease. The histological findings suggestive of coeliac disease are villous atrophy, intra-epithelial white cell infiltration and crypt hyperplasia. Multiple biopsies should be taken, as there can be patchy involvement. The treatment of coeliac disease relies on lifelong adherence to a gluten-free diet.

Green PHR and Cellier C. Celiac Disease. The New England Journal of Medicine. 2007;357: 1731-43

9) B: Appendix

This patient has a carcinoid tumour. It is a serotonin-secreting tumour of the enterochromaffin cells most commonly arising in the appendix. The serotonin released from the appendiceal carcinoid tumour enters the portal circulation and is largely metabolised by the liver. However, once the tumour spreads to the liver, high levels of serotonin enters the systemic circulation causing features of the carcinoid syndrome, which span diarrhoea, paroxysmal facial flushing and bronchial wheeze. The principal metabolite of serotonin, 5-hydroxyindoleacetic acid is elevated in the syndrome.

Zuetenhorst JM and Taal BG. Metastatic Carcinoid Tumours: A Clinical Review. The Oncologist. 2005;10: 123-31

10) C: Gastrografin swallow

The most likely diagnosis is Boerhaave's syndrome, defined by spontaneous oesophageal perforation following straining, retching or vomiting. The occurrence of severe, central chest or epigastric pain following vomiting should immediately raise suspicion of this diagnosis due its high mortality rate. Patients frequently develop mediastinitis, sepsis and multiorgan dysfunction.

The presence of subcutaneous emphysema (accounting for the crackling feeling on palpation) is present in up to 60% of patients but occurs at least 1 hour after perforation, whilst 50% of patients present with Mackler's triad (vomiting, chest pain and subcutaneous emphysema).

The leading cause of oesophageal perforation is iatrogenic accounting for 70% of cases.

Kaman L, Iqbal J, Kandil B and Kochhar R. Management of Esophageal Perforation in Adults. Gastroenterology Research. 2010;3: 235-44

11) C: Vitamin B3

This patient has pellagra, which is characterised by the 4Ds: Dermatitis, diarrhoea, dementia and death. It is a rare condition caused by niacin (vitamin B3) deficiency. Patients susceptible to pellagra include chronic alcoholics, those with malabsorption states and food faddists. The rash in pellagra is a bilaterally, symmetrical, photosensitive rash occurring in sun-exposed areas. When around the neck, the rash is quite characteristic in that it can resemble a broad necklace ('Casal's necklace'). Psychiatric manifestations are legion and span depression, mania, delusions, hallucinations, anxiety and irritability. In severe cases, patients develop dementia, eventually entering into a coma and dying, unless treated early. Mucosal inflammation and atrophy leads to malabsorption and diarrhoea. Patients frequently complain of poor appetite, nausea, vomiting and abdominal discomfort. Due to the relatively non-specific gastrointestinal symptoms, making the diagnosis requires a high index of suspicion and the ability to recognise the pattern of symptoms and signs spanning the different organ systems.

Vitamin A deficiency can lead to xeropthalmia, night blindness and visual loss.
Vitamin B1 (thiamine) deficiency leads to beriberi syndrome.
Vitamin B2 (riboflavin) deficiency frequently causes angular stomatitis and glossitis.
Vitamin B6 (pyridoxine) deficiency leads to peripheral neuropathy.
Vitamin B9 (folate) and B12 deficiency can cause megaloblastic anaemia.
Vitamin C deficiency results in scurvy.

Hegyi J, Schwartz RA and Hegyi V. Pellagra: Dermatitis, dementia and diarrhoea. International Journal of Dermatology. 2004;43: 1-5.

12) D: Penicillamine

The diagnosis is Wilson's disease, which is caused by a mutation in the ATP7B gene on chromosome 13. This mutation compromises the function of a copper transporting protein required to facilitate hepatocellular excretion of copper into the bile. Presentation during childhood is thus in the form of hepatitis, liver failure and cirrhosis owing to the abnormal accumulation of copper in the liver. Copper can also accumulate in the basal ganglia and lead to neurological sequelae, which include Parkinsonism, neuropsychiatric manifestations, dysarthria, dysphagia, dystonia and tremor (classically a wing-beating tremor). Presentation of such CNS features is usually in young adults who have already developed features of liver failure. Investigation findings include elevated 24-hour urinary copper excretion (> 100 micrograms) and low serum caeruloplasmin levels.

Treatment involves lifelong penicillamine therapy and ultimately liver transplantation in those with end-stage liver cirrhosis.

Roberts EA and Schilsky ML. Diagnosis and Treatment of Wilson Disease: An Update. Hepatology. 2008;47: 2089-111.

13) A: Omeprazole, amoxicillin and clarithromycin

Helicobacter pylori infection represents the single biggest risk factor for the formation of peptic ulcers. It is more strongly associated with duodenal than gastric ulcers, representing the aetiology in 90% and up to 80% of cases, respectively.

The rapid urease test is an invasive test for H.pylori, applied on biopsy specimens and relies on the production of urease by the bacteria, which converts urea to ammonia, raising the pH and causing a colour change on a pH indicator.

Eradicating H.pylori via triple therapy (e.g. 1 week course of omeprazole, amoxicillin and clarithromycin, or omeprazole, metronidazole and clarithromycin) is the most reliable means of treating and preventing recurrence of peptic ulceration.

McColl KEL. Helicobacter Pylori Infection. The New England Journal of Medicine. 2010;362: 1597-1604

14) E: Gram-negative facultative anaerobic bacilli

The diagnosis is spontaneous bacterial peritonitis (SBP), which is recognised as a severe complication of ascites secondary to liver cirrhosis. It is thought to occur as a consequence of bacterial translocation from the gut lumen into the peritoneal cavity due to increased small bowel permeability, explaining why gut flora micro-organisms account for the majority of causes. E.coli represents the commonest infective aetiology (Klebsiella being the second commonest). Although patients typically present with abdominal pain, varying from mild to severe with peritonism, its absence does not exclude the diagnosis. Other features that should raise suspicion of SBP include signs and symptoms of sepsis, especially where no other source is identified, and features of liver decompensation, such as worsening ascites refractory to diuretic therapy, hepatic encephalopathy, coagulopathy and general deterioration.

The diagnosis is confirmed by an ascitic tap, which shows a neutrophil count of more than 250 cells/microliter.

Guidelines from the American Association for the study of liver diseases recommend third generation cephalosporins, preferably intravenous cefotaxime as first-line antibiotic therapy.

Lata J, Stiburek O and Kopacova M. Spontaneous bacterial peritonitis: A severe complication of liver cirrhosis. World Journal of Gastroenterology. 2009;15: 5505-5510

15) A: C-13 urea breath test and H. Pylori eradication, if positive

This patient presents with dyspepsia, a common complaint amongst the general population. Presentation is vague with abdominal discomfort, nausea and bloating and can potentially be due to multiple aetiologies, including gastritis, peptic ulceration and gastro-oesophageal reflux disease (GORD).

Patients with new-onset dyspepsia who are more than 55 years of age and/or present with the so-called 'alarm' symptoms (such as *unexplained weight loss, bleeding, anaemia, persistent vomiting, dysphagia or lymphadenopathy* to name a few) should undergo an urgent oesophago-gastro-duodenoscopy (OGD) to exclude more sinister possibilities such as upper GI malignancy. The patient's age and absence of such alarm features makes option B) incorrect.

Guidelines from the American Journal of Gastroenterology have recommended the test and treat strategy (option A) in areas where the prevalence of H.Pylori infection is more than 10%. If the prevalence were less than 10%, then a 4 to 8 week trial of PPI would have been more appropriate.

The urea breath test is the most accurate non-invasive test for diagnosing H. pylori infection with a sensitivity of 95% and specificity of 98%. The test exists in two forms (C13 and C14 urea breath tests) and involves drinking a solution containing urea labelled with C13 (or C14). It relies on the production of urease by H.pylori, which splits the urea and releases the correspondingly labelled carbon dioxide. The levels of C13 (or C14) labelled carbon dioxide correlates with the intensity of urease enzyme activity and the degree of H. pylori colonisation.

Braden B. Diagnosis of Helicobacter pylori infection. British Medical Journal. 2012;344: e828

Talley NJ, Vakil N; Practise Parameters Committee of the American College of Gastroenterology. American Journal of Gastroenterology. 2005;100: 2324-37.

16) B: 750-1500ml

Less than 15% of circulating blood volume lost (Approx 750mls) usually results in an increased respiratory rate and occasionally a mild tachycardia with a normal blood pressure.

Loss of 15-30% of circulating volume (750-1500mls) results in a tachycardia and normal or low/normal blood pressure.

20-40% loss (1500-2000mls) results in a tachycardia, hypotension and occasionally confusion

>40% blood loss (>2000mls) can result in a critically low blood pressure and requires aggressive intervention.

Scottish Intercollegiate Guidelines Network. Management of acute upper and lower gastrointestinal bleeding. CG 105. 2008.

17) E: Peutz-Jegher's syndrome

This patient has presented with symptoms and signs of acute bowel obstruction secondary to intussusception. The most likely underlying cause for this, given the perioral and buccal pigmentation, is Peutz-Jeghers syndrome (PJS).

This is a rare, autosomal dominant condition, characterised by a combination of mucocutaneous hyperpigmentation and the development of multiple hamartomatous polyps throughout the gastrointestinal (GI) tract. Patients commonly present with a history of recurrent colicky abdominal pain, which may culminate in intussuception and accompanying bowel obstruction.

Although hamartomatous polyps may undergo neoplastic transformation resulting in an increased risk of bowel cancer, patients with PJS are also at higher risk of other malignancies including pancreatic, lung, liver, breast and testicular cancer.

Lynch syndrome is also known as hereditary non-polyposis colon cancer (HNPCC) and does not produce the clinical picture described. Although patients with familial adenomatous polyposis may rarely present with intussusception, they lack the perioral and buccal hyperpigmentation that characterises PJS.

Thakker HH, Joshi A and Deshpande A. Peutz-Jegher's syndrome presenting as jejunoileal intussusception in an adult male: a case report. Cases Journal. 2009;2: 8865

Utsunomiya J, Gocho H, Miyanaga T, Hamaguchi E and Kashimure A. Peutz-Jeghers syndrome: its natural course and management. The John Hopkins Medical Journal. 1975;136: 71-82

18) A: Intravenous bolus of omeprazole 80mg followed by an infusion of 8mg/hour

Management of bleeding peptic ulcer disease requires 2 forms of endo-therapy. If therapy is administered, proton pump inhibition should be maintained intravenously for 72hours.

Gralnek IM, Barkun AN and Bardou M. Management of Acute Bleeding from a Peptic Ulcer. The New England Journal of Medicine. 2008;359: 928-37.

19) D: Propanolol

Patients with liver cirrhosis develop portal hypertension as a consequence of:

1) *Increased intrahepatic resistance* - this occurs as a result of microarchitectural distortion of the liver secondary to fibrosis and nodular regeneration and active intrahepatic vasoconstriction.
2) *Increased portal in-flow* – secondary to splanchnic arteriolar vasodilatation

Increased portal pressures induce the formation of porto-systemic anastomotic venous shunts, of which oesophageal varices are an example. Despite these shunts, however, portal pressures remain high as a consequence of maintained splanchic vasodilatation and the high resistance of the collateral venous channels.

Non-selective beta-blockers, such as propanolol have been shown to halve the risk of variceal bleeds (from 30% to 15%) in cirrhotic patients. They function by inducing splanchic vasoconstriction and reducing cardiac output, which collectively contribute to reducing portal venous pressures.

Although terlipressin and vasopressin drive splanchic vasoconstriction, their use is reserved in the management of acute variceal bleeding and not in primary prophylaxis.

Garcia-Tsao G, Sanyal AJ, Grace ND, Carey W; Practise Guidelines Committee of the American Association for the Study of Liver Diseases; Practise Parameters Committee of the American College of Gastroenterology. Hepatology. 2007;46: 922-38

20) C: Delta cells

21) E: CA 19-9

The development of painless jaundice in an elderly patient signifies pancreatic cancer until proven otherwise. The other ominous feature in the history is unintentional weight loss, which further raises suspicion of malignancy. Conjugated hyperbilirubinaemia, which occurs in obstructive jaundice, is responsible for producing dark urine. Under normal circumstances bilirubin is excreted as part of the bile pigment via the bile ducts into the intestines. In the large bowel, bilirubin is then normally converted into urobilinogen and then into stercobilin, which gives the stool its brown colour. In obstructive jaundice, there is a lack of stercobilin formation in the large bowel and therefore the stool becomes pale in colour.

Raised levels of CA 19-9 is classically associated with pancreatic cancer, AFP with hepatocellular carcinoma, CEA with colon cancer, hCG with germ cell tumours and CA 125 with ovarian carcinoma. However, these associations are not completely specific as for example, CA 19-9 can also be elevated in some cases of colorectal cancer.

Hidalgo M. Pancreatic Cancer. The New England Journal of Medicine. 2010;362: 1605-17

22) A: Whipple's disease

Fenollar F, Puechal X and Raoult D. Whipple's Disease. The New England Journal of Medicine. 2007;356: 55-66.

23) C: Thumbprinting

Sentinel loop sign indicates localised ileus secondary to local inflammation, most commonly seen in conditions such as acute pancreatitis.

The string sign is seen in contrast x-rays in conditions such as Crohn's Disease, Carcinoid and Colon Cancer and is due to structuring.

The corkscrew sign as the name suggests is associated with volvulus.

24) B: Alcohol excess

An AST/ALT ratio of >2.0 is most commonly associated with alcohol hepatitis.

25) E: Acute mesenteric ischaemia

The preceding symptoms of abdominal migraine precipitated by food intake are highly suggestive of pre-existing chronic mesenteric ischaemia. Mesenteric Angiography is diagnostic for this condition. Management involves lifestyle and pharmacological optimisation of vascular risk factors although it may be possible to stent or bypass occluded mesenteric vessels.

Acute mesenteric occlusion, however, presents acutely and can occur on a background of underlying mesenteric vascular disease, or result from embolic disease in the absence of preceding abdominal migraine.

The clues in this case, which are suggestive of mesenteric ischaemia, are the rectal bleeding and a background of vascular risk factors. Most acute abdominal pathologies can cause an elevated amylase and lactate, however an extremely elevated lactate is more commonly associated with ischaemic phenomena.

26) E: Mallory-Weiss tear

27) C: Achalasia

28) D: Metronidazole

Giardia lamblia is an anaerobic flagellated protozoan, which is usually acquired from contaminated food, soil or water. Symptoms often include violent diarrhoea and abdominal cramps. Typically, infection lasts 2-6 weeks. Metronidazole reduces symptoms and time to resolution.

29) C: DQ2

HLA DR3 is associated with myasthenia gravis, Hashimoto's thyroiditis and Primary Sclerosing Cholangitis.

HLA DR4 is associated with rheumatoid arthritis and systemic lupus erytematosus.

HLA DQ8 is associated with Coeliac Disease, Rheumatoid Arthritis and Juvenile Arthritis

HLA B27 is best known for its association with seronegative spondyloarthropathies such as Ankylosing Spondylitis.

Yuan Y, Padol IT and Hunt RH. Peptic ulcer disease today. Nature Clinical Practise Gastroenterology & Hepatology. 2006;3: 80-9.

30) E: Rectal Carcinoma

The presence of unintentional weight loss, and change in bowel habit should always alert the examining clinician towards a diagnosis of malignancy. Ischaemic colitis is usually associated with pain and symptoms of postprandial abdominal pain. Although proton pump inhibitors are associated with an increased risk of Clostridium difficile diarrhoea, this is usually bloodless.

31) D: CT scan

Large passage of blood per-rectally should always be investigated. Previously documented evidence of diverticulae does not exclude other diagnoses. In a frail patient with poor mobility, the risks associated with bowel preparation need to be weighed up against a less invasive and equally effective diagnostic imaging such as CT scans.

32) D: Diverticulosis is the commonest cause of massive haematochezia

Massive rectal bleeding is associated with diverticulosis in approximately 50% of cases. The mere presence of diverticulae with no evidence of inflammation or bleeding is not a cause for Iron deficiency, and alternative aetiologies should be considered. Diverticular associated colitis has been documented to recur even after resection. There is no association between Meckels and colonic diverticulosis.

33) A: Obesity is a risk factor for diverticular bleeding

A BMI >30 is associated with an increased risk of diverticular bleeding. Whilst lethargy can be associated with diverticular disease, its presence is usually seen in older patients with Irritable Bowel Syndrome, and other gastrointestinal symptoms suggestive of fistula formation or bleeding are more commonly reported. Diverticular associated colitis is considered a separate entity to Inflammatory Bowel Disease.

Whilst 5'ASA drugs are the mainstay of treatment, there is no role for steroids.

34) A: The earliest time a reliable plasma paracetamol level can be measured is 8 hours after the time of overdose

The earliest time a reliable plasma paracetamol level can be measured is 4 hours after the time of overdose. However in a significant paracetamol overdose, or unclear history of quantity or timing of overdose, N-Acetylcysteine should not be delayed with or without plasma paracetamol levels.

35) B: Gilbert's syndrome

Dubin-Johnson syndrome causes a conjugated hyperbilirubinaemia, whereas Gilbert's syndrome leads to an unconjugated hyperbilirubinaemia.

36) D: Oral metronidazole for 10 days

Oral, not intravenous, vancomycin is the alternative (or supplementary) treatment for C. Diff colitis.

37) E: Digoxin

Calcium channel blockers, anticholinergics, nitrates and tricyclic antidepressants are all associated with relaxation of the lower oesophageal sphincter and therefore predispose to gastro-oesophageal reflux disease.

Digoxin has little effect on lower oeseophageal sphincter pressures and is therefore the correct answer.

38) D: 6

The most likely diagnosis is hereditary haemochromatosis.

39) E: A normal endoscopy excludes a diagnosis of GORD

40) B: Laparoscopic resection with end-end anastomosis is always the preferred management strategy

Complicated diverticulitis with fistula formation is unlikely to resolve with medical management.

Surgical therapy is the preferred management option, but evidence for a laparoscopic approach has demonstrated best results in larger experienced centres, and is usually preferred after the acute phase is over. There is no evidence that age be a factor in directing laparoscopic versus open surgery.

The presence of a pelvic abscess suggests a need for a surgical or radiological drainage procedure as they almost never improve without intervention.

Nephrology Questions

1) A 68-year old gentleman is seen in the nephrology clinic. An ultrasound KUB has shown a right kidney measuring 10.4cm and a left kidney measuring 6.5cm, longitudinally.

   Past medical history includes chronic obstructive pulmonary disease and peripheral vascular disease.

   On examination, abdomen is soft, non-tender, and a left carotid bruit is audible.

   What is the next most appropriate investigation required to make a diagnosis?

   A. CT KUB
   B. Renal biopsy
   C. Magnetic resonance angiography
   D. Intravenous urogram
   E. 24 hour urine collection

2) A 32-year old male develops severe flank pain. He reports that his father and grandfather suffered with kidney trouble, which eventually required dialysis. An ultrasound KUB is performed, which shows bilaterally enlarged kidneys with numerous multiple cysts.

   Which of the following is most strongly associated with this condition?

   A. Mitral valve stenosis
   B. Mitral valve prolapse
   C. Aortic regurgitation
   D. Aortic stenosis
   E. Tricuspid valve stenosis

3) A 48-year old female presents to the emergency department with severe, colicky right loin pain radiating to her groin.

   A renal calculus is identified on CT KUB.

What is the most likely composition of this in the general population?

A. Uric acid
B. Cystine
C. Calcium Oxalate
D. Magnesium ammonium phosphate
E. Calcium Hydroxyapatite

4) A 24-year old male presents to the assessment unit with macroscopic haematuria 2 days after developing a sore throat.

Urine microscopy shows red cell casts.

What is the most likely diagnosis?

A. Membranous nephropathy
B. Mesangiocapillary glomerulonephritis
C. Post-streptococcal glomerulonephritis
D. Berger's disease
E. Minimal change glomerulonephritis

5) A 28-year old female presents under the medical take with severe left-sided loin pain.

Urine dipstick shows haematuria +++.

An abdominal X-ray is undertaken which reveals a staghorn calculus.

What micro-organism is the urine most likely to culture?

A. Eschericia Coli
B. Proteus Mirabilis
C. Klebsiella pneumoniae
D. Staphylococcus Saprophyticus
E. Ureaplasma Urealyticum

6) A 4-year old boy is brought to clinic because of facial and lower limb oedema.

A 24-hour urine collection confirms nephrotic-range proteinuria.

Which of the following statements regarding microscopy of a renal biopsy specimen from this patient is most likely to be true?

A. Fusion of the podocyte foot processes on electron microscopy
B. Thickened glomerular basement membrane visible on light microscopy
C. Tram-line appearance on the basement membrane under light microscopy
D. Global scarring of the glomeruli under light microscopy
E. Normal appearance on electron microscopy

7) Which of the following correctly describes the effects of ramipril on the glomerular apparatus?

A. Relative constriction of the efferent arteriole
B. Relative constriction of the afferent arteriole
C. Relative dilatation of the efferent arteriole
D. Relative dilatation of the afferent arteriole
E. Equal constriction of the afferent and efferent arteriole

8) A 42-year old lady presents with bilateral lower limb swelling with pitting oedema to the mid-shins.

24-hour urinary protein excretion is 3.5 g and serum albumin is 18.

What is the most likely underlying pathological cause for her clinical presentation?

A. Minimal change nephropathy
B. Focal segmental glomerulosclerosis
C. Mesangiocapillary glomerulonephritis
D. IgA nephropathy
E. Membranous nephropathy

9) Which of the following is NOT an indication for urgent haemodialysis in patients with acute kidney injury?

A. An increase in creatinine to more than 500 micromol/l
B. Pulmonary oedema
C. Uraemic pericarditis
D. Hyperkalaemia refractory to medical treatment
E. Severe metabolic acidosis (pH < 7.2)

10) A 65-year old male presents with 3-day history of diarrhoea and vomiting to the acute medical take.

He is known to have chronic kidney disease with a baseline creatinine of around 130 micromol/l.

On examination, he has dry mucous membranes and reduced skin turgor. Heart rate is 80/min regular and blood pressure is 128/76 mmHg.

Investigations show:

Na	149	(135-145mmol/l)
K	6.8	(3.5-5mmol/l)
Urea	19.6	(2.2-8.3mmol/l)
Creat	320	(60-100micromol/l)

12-lead ECG: sinus rhythm, tented T-waves and broad QRS complexes

What is the first most appropriate management?

A. Urgent haemodialysis
B. Intravenous fluid resuscitation
C. 5mg salbutamol nebulisers stat
D. 10 units intravenous actrapid in 50ml 50% dextrose over 30 minutes
E. 10 ml of 10% intravenous calcium gluconate

11) A 76-year old patient with CKD stage 5 is reviewed in clinic.

Her most recent blood results reveal:

Serum calcium   1.84   (2.20-2.60 mmol/L)

Serum phosphate   1.50   (0.80-1.45 mmol/L)

PTH   16.2   (0.8-8.5 pmol/L)

What is the most likely diagnosis?

A. Primary hyperparathyroidism
B. Secondary hyperparathyroidism
C. Tertiary hyperparathyroidism
D. Vitamin D deficiency
E. Pseudo-hypoparathyroidism

12) A patient known to have chronic kidney disease (CKD) is reviewed in clinic. His most recent estimated glomerular filtration rate (eGFR) is 50 ml/min/1.73m².

What stage CKD does he have?

A. Stage 1
B. Stage 2
C. Stage 3
D. Stage 4
E. Stage 5

13) Which of the following statements correctly describes the pathophysiology underlying type 1 renal tubular acidosis?

A. Failure of the proximal tubule to secrete hydrogen ions
B. Failure of the proximal tubule to reabsorb bicarbonate ions
C. Failure of the distal tubule to secrete hydrogen ions
D. Failure of the distal tubule to reabsorb bicarbonate ions
E. Metabolic acidosis secondary to hyporeninaemic hypoaldosteronism

14) A 68-year old lady is diagnosed with acute kidney injury secondary to sepsis. A urine sample is sent to biochemistry for various tests.

Which of the following results is suggestive of acute tubular necrosis as opposed to pre-renal kidney injury?

A. Urine osmolarity of 540 mOsm/l
B. Urine sodium of 50 mmol/l
C. Fractional sodium excretion of 0.4%
D. Urine/plasma urea ratio of 10
E. Urine/plasma creatinine ratio of 60

15) A 48-year old female was recently started on penicillin for a sore throat. One week later, she developed arthralgia (for which she took paracetamol and ibuprofen), fevers and rash. She is otherwise fit and well with no significant past medical history. Bloods show:

Hb	12.8 g/dl
White cells	10.3×10^9/L
Neutrophils	4.4×10^9/L
Eosinophils	5.2×10^9/L
Basophils	0.2×10^9/L

Na^+	138 mmol/l
K^+	5.0 mmol/l
Urea	18.0 mmol/l
Creat	220 micromol/l

What is the most likely diagnosis?

A. Acute tubular necrosis
B. Analgesic nephropathy
C. Balkan nephropathy
D. Post-streptococcal glomerulonephritis
E. Acute tubulo-interstitial nephritis

16) A patient takes amiloride for congestive cardiac failure.

What is the mechanism of action of this drug?

A. Blocks the Na-K-2Cl co-transporter in the thick ascending limb of the Loop of Henle
B. Inhibits carbonic anhydrase
C. Blocks the Na-Cl co-transport in the distal convoluted tubule
D. Antagonises the aldosterone receptor in the cortical collecting duct
E. Blocks the epithelial Na channel in the distal tubule and collecting ducts

17) An 18-year old female is brought to the emergency department with a 3-day history of dysuria and frequency.

On examination, she looks generally unwell and sweaty and has significant left-sided flank tenderness.
Observations are: heart rate 120/min regular, blood pressure 88/60 mmHg and temperature 38.6 degrees.

Urine dipstick shows leukocytes 3+ and nitrites +.

Which of the following is the first most appropriate management?

A. Intravenous co-amoxiclav
B. Stat dose of intravenous gentamicin
C. Ultrasound KUB
D. Fluid challenge with 500ml gelofusine
E. Urgent bloods with blood cultures

18) Which of the following statements concerning renal physiology is incorrect?

A. Renin is secreted by the juxtaglomerular apparatus
B. Hyperkalaemia directly increases aldosterone secretion from the zona glomerulosa
C. Renal blood flow corresponds to nearly 15% of cardiac output
D. Osmolarity increases towards the medulla
E. Anti-diuretic hormone increases the number of aquaporin-2 channels in the collecting duct apical membranes

19) The results from an MSU sent from a woman who is 13-weeks pregnant returns as:

Growth of E. coli > 100, 000 organisms per ml, sensitivities pending

She denies any recent history of dysuria, frequency or urgency and feels completely well in herself.

What is the most appropriate management?

A. As she is asymptomatic, no further treatment is necessary
B. Repeat MSU in 2 weeks time, and if positive, commence antibiotics
C. Repeat MSU in 4 weeks time, and if positive, commence antibiotics
D. Give a 3-day course of trimethoprim, unless contraindicated
E. Give a 5-day course of co-amoxiclav, unless contraindicated

20) A 28-year old male presents with a 1-week history of haematuria. He also reports increasing shortness of breath lately and coughing up blood-tinged sputum.

Chest X-ray reveals bilateral patchy infiltrates.

What is the most likely diagnosis?

A. Young's syndrome
B. Alport's syndrome
C. Tietze's syndrome
D. Goodpasture's syndrome
E. Sarcoidosis

Nephrology Answers

1) C: Magnetic resonance angiography

The combination of peripheral vascular disease and objective evidence of arteriosclerotic disease (carotid bruit) increases the risk of renal artery stenosis, of which the most common cause is atherosclerosis. This suspicion is further raised by the fact that ultrasound KUB has demonstrated asymmetry in the sizes of both kidneys. Magnetic resonance angiography is the most reliable non-invasive investigation that can be employed to diagnose renal artery stenosis.

2) B: Mitral valve prolapse

This patient has autosomal dominant polycystic kidney disease (ADPKD), which affects nearly 1 in 800 live births. Patients develop multiple renal cysts bilaterally and most commonly present in the 30-50 year age range with flank or lower back pain (e.g. as a result of haemorrhage into a cyst or cyst rupture), hypertension, haematuria, recurrent urinary tract infections and renal calculi. It is incurable and inexorably leads to end stage renal failure by the age of 60 in half of patients.

ADPKD is caused by a mutation in the polycystin 1 (chromosome 16), and polycystin 2 (chromosome 4) genes, in 85% and 15% of cases, respectively. Very rarely PKD is inherited in an autosomal recessive fashion, but has a very much distinct phenotype, frequently presenting in the neonatal period.

ADPKD is strongly associated with various extra-renal manifestations including berry aneurysms (look out for a family history of subarachnoid haemorrhage), mitral valve prolapse and liver cysts. Mitral valve prolapse is also associated with Marfans's syndrome, rheumatoid arthritis, Turner's syndrome and ankylosing spondylitis.

Wilson PD. Polycystic Kidney Disease. The New England Journal of Medicine. 2004;350: 151-64.

3) C: Calcium Oxalate

The classical clinic presentation of renal calculi is severe, sudden onset, colicky pain, radiating from the loin to the groin, alongside haematuria (though this may be microscopic). The most common composition is calcium oxalate, unless the calculus is of the staghorn type, in which case magnesium ammonium phosphate is more likely.

4) D: Berger's disease

Berger's disease (IgA nephropathy) is the most common cause of glomerulonephritis worldwide. It presents as macroscopic (or microscopic) haematuria 1-3 days after an upper respiratory tract infection. Although post-streptococcal glomerulonephritis is a tempting answer, this characteristically presents 10-14 days after a sore throat.

5) B: Proteus Mirabilis

Although E. Coli is the most common cause of urinary tract infections, Proteus represents the most common cause of complicated UTIs that result in the formation of staghorn calculi. The composition of this urinary tract stone is Magnesium Ammonium Phosphate and is also referred to as the 'triple phosphate' stone.

6) A: Fusion of the podocyte foot processes on electron microscopy

Nephrotic syndrome is characterised by:

1) Heavy proteinuria (> 3-3.5g/24 hours or a spot protein: creatinine ratio of > 300-350 mg/mmol)
2) Oedema
3) Hypoalbuminaemia (albumin < 25 g/l)
4) Hyperlipidaemia (total cholesterol often > 10mmol/l)

Patients with nephrotic syndrome are at high risk of thromboembolism (as a result of urinary losses of antithrombin III), thereby necessitating thromboprophylaxis, and infection.

The most common cause of nephrotic syndrome in children is minimal-change glomerulonephropathy. The name is derived from the fact that under light microscopy, renal biopsy specimens show normal-looking glomeruli. However, under the electron microscope, there is usually evidence of fusion of the podocyte foot processes, hence option A is the correct answer. Most children (95%) enter remission with steroid therapy, but poor response may require use of steroid-sparing agents like cyclophosphamide.

Orth SR and Ritz E. The Nephrotic Syndrome. The New England Journal of Medicine. 1998;338: 1202-1211

7) C: Relative dilatation of the efferent arteriole

The glomerular filtration rate (GFR) is driven by a difference in blood flow through the afferent and efferent arterioles. Dilatation of the afferent arteriole and constriction of the efferent arteriole collectively create a gradient in flow rates across the glomerulus, which helps increase the GFR. Afferent arteriolar dilatation is mediated by prostaglandins, whilst efferent arteriolar constriction is mediated by angiotensin II. The relative balance of prostaglandin and angiotensin II activity is a key process that determines the magnitude of the GFR (although in reality, a host of other mediators operate in influencing and fine-tuning the GFR).

Non-steroidal anti-inflammatory drugs (NSAIDs) inhibit prostaglandin synthesis and therefore induce a relative constriction of the afferent arteriole. ACE inhibitors and angiotensin II receptor blockers (A2RBs), which reduce angiotensin II synthesis or activity, respectively, cause a relative dilatation of the efferent arteriole. Thus, NSAIDs and ACE inhibitors/A2RBs both reduce GFR via distinct mechanisms.

8) E. Membranous nephropathy

The clinical presentation is nephrotic syndrome and in adults, the most common cause is membranous nephropathy. Membranous nephropathy can arise secondary to many different conditions including diabetes, drugs (especially captopril, gold, penicillamine) and connective tissue disease (e.g. SLE) but is idiopathic in the majority of patients.

Hull RP and Goldsmith DJA. Nephrotic syndrome in adults. British Medical Journal. 2008;336: 1185-9

9) A: An increase in creatinine to more than 500 micromol/l

A significant increase in creatinine is not in itself an indication for urgent haemodialysis. The following describe the recognised indications for urgent haemodialysis in acute kidney injury:

1) Symptomatic uraemia (e.g. uraemic pericarditis, uraemic encephalopathy)
2) Refractory hyperkalaemia (potassium more than 7mmol/l) despite medical treatment
3) Severe metabolic acidosis (pH< 7.2)
4) Pulmonary oedema

10) E: 10 ml of 10% intravenous calcium gluconate

This patient presents with an acute-on-chronic kidney injury secondary to dehydration as a result of D and V. The causes of acute kidney injury (AKI) can be divided into:

1) *Pre-renal*: hypovolaemia (e.g. blood loss, dehydration, burns, sepsis)
2) *Renal*: acute tubular necrosis secondary to drugs, ischaemic damage, vasculitis, contrast agents
3) *Post-renal*: obstructive uropathies

Dehydration can lead to a pre-renal kidney injury as a result of generalised afferent arteriolar constriction and a consequently globally reduced glomerular filtration rate. In severe cases, this can lead to hyperkalaemia, metabolic acidosis, symptomatic uraemia and potentially pulmonary oedema.

This patient has significant hyperkalaemia with corresponding hyperkalaemic ECG changes (hyperkalaemia should be actively treated if the potassium is more than 6.5 mmol/l or if there are ECG changes). Hyperkalaemic ECG changes include tall tented T-waves, prolonged QRS complexes, small or absent p-waves with prolonged PR intervals, which if left untreated, can potentially deteriorate into ventricular fibrillation or asystole; significant hyperkalaemia is therefore a medical emergency necessitating urgent treatment.

Although intravenous fluid resuscitation represents an essential component of the management of pre-renal AKI, this answer is incorrect, as the hyperkalaemia must be addressed first (in reality, patients are given IV fluid resuscitation simultaneously). Intravenous calcium gluconate does not affect potassium levels, but is cardioprotective and buys time for further management. This should be followed by an IV infusion of 10 units actrapid in dextrose over 30 minutes, which lowers potassium by 1 mmol/l and its effects last for around 1-2 hours. Salbutamol nebulisers can help further lower potassium.

11) B: Secondary hyperparathyroidism

Patients with CKD are liable to secondary hyperparathyroidism. High PTH levels arise because of a combination of reduced activation of vitamin D3, hypocalcaemia and hyperphosphataemia (which further exacerbates hypocalcaemia) in CKD. The compromised vitamin D3 activation occurs because of reduced 1-alpha hydroxylase activity, which leads to a reduced production of 1,25-dihydroxycholecalciferol from 25-hydroxycholecalciferol. When secondary hyperparathyroidism becomes prolonged, the parathyroid glands begin to autonomously secrete PTH, leading to a tertiary hyperparathyroidism, manifesting as hyper- or normocalcaemia.

Secondary hyperparathyroidism predisposes patients to osteitis fibrosa cystica, a major form of renal bone disease characterised by increased resorption of bone, largely owing to raised osteoclast activity driven by high PTH levels. Adynamic bone disease is another form of renal bone disease and is a result of reduced PTH levels, commonly an iatrogenic result of excessive calcium and vitamin D consumption.

Tomasello S. Secondary Hyperparathyroidism and Chronic Kidney Disease. Diabetes Spectrum. 2008;21: 19-25

Martin KJ and Gonzalez EA. Metabolic Bone Disease in Chronic Kidney Disease. Journal of the American Society of Nephrology. 2007; 18: 875-85

12) C: Stage 3

Chronic kidney disease (CKD) can be divided into stages according to the eGFR (in ml/min/$1.73m^2$) as shown below:

Stage 1: > 90 ml/min/$1.73m^2$, with other evidence of kidney damage
Stage 2: 60-90 ml/min/$1.73m^2$, with other evidence of kidney damage
Stage 3A: 45-60 ml/min/$1.73m^2$, with or without evidence of kidney damage
Stage 3B: 30-45 ml/min/$1.73m^2$, with or without evidence of kidney damage
Stage 4: 15-30 ml/min/$1.73m^2$, with or without evidence of kidney damage
Stage 5: < 15 ml/min/$1.73m^2$; end-stage renal failure

(Evidence of kidney damage includes persistent proteinuria, albuminuria, haematuria or pathological structural abnormalities of the kidneys).

Risk factors for CKD include diabetes mellitus, hypertension, cardiovascular disease, smoking, family history of CKD and connective tissue diseases. Controlling the risk factors that can be controlled should help slow down the progression of CKD. Unlike acute kidney injury, ACE inhibitors play a central role in slowing down the progression of CKD by reducing proteinuria.

According to NICE guidelines, the following patients should be offered ACE inhibitors:

1) Patients with hypertension and proteinuria (albumin: creatinine ratio > 30mg/mmol, protein:creatinine ratio > 50mg/mmol or a urinary protein excretion > 0.5g/24)
2) Patients without hypertension but heavier proteinuria (albumin: creatinine ratio >70mg/mmol, protein:creatinine ratio > 100mg/mmol or a urinary protein excretion > 1g/24)
3) Diabetic patients with microalbuminuria

Patients with CKD are generally asymptomatic until they progress to end-stage renal failure where they become significantly uraemic (nowadays patients are usually offered renal replacement therapy before this happens). Patients with CKD stage 5 develop:

1) Weight loss, cachexia and weakness
2) Anaemia –anaemia of chronic disease and a lack of erythropoietin production
3) Renal osteodystrophy – mainly spanning osteitis fibrosia cystica and adynamic bone disease
4) Uraemia - which can lead to pericarditis, platelet dysfunction, peripheral neuropathy, gastrointestinal symptoms such as nausea, vomiting and diarrhoea, skin dryness and pruritus, confusion and encephalopathy

National Institute for Health and Clinical Excellence. 2008. CG73. Chronic kidney disease: Early identification and management of chronic kidney disease in adults in primary and secondary care. London: National Institute for Health and Clinical Excellence.

Levey AS and Coresh J. Chronic kidney disease. Lancet. 2012; 379: 165-80

13) C: Failure of the distal tubule to secrete hydrogen ions

Type 1 renal tubular acidosis (RTA), also known as distal renal tubular acidosis, is an important cause of metabolic acidosis with a normal anion gap. It occurs as a result of failure of the distal renal tubule to secrete sufficient hydrogen ions despite a metabolic acidaemia. The diagnosis is made if the urine remains inappropriately alkaline (pH > 5.5) despite an oral acid load like ammonium chloride.

Type 1 RTA is often idiopathic but can be associated with multiple conditions including nephrocalcinosis, SLE, chronic pyelonephritis and drugs like lithium.

Type 2 RTA, also known as proximal RTA, is caused by a failure of the proximal tubule to reabsorb sufficient bicarbonate anions. This frequently occurs as part of a more global defect in proximal tubular reabsorptive function (e.g. Fanconi syndrome)

Metabolic acidosis secondary to hyporeninaemic hypoaldosteronism characterises type 4 RTA.

Unwin RJ and Capasso G. The renal tubular acidoses. Journal of the Royal Society of Medicine. 2001;94: 221-25

14) **B: Urine sodium of 50 mmol/l**

Acute tubular necrosis (ATN) represents the commonest renal cause of AKI. The death of tubular cells in the nephrons compromise the concentrating ability of the kidneys in ATN, whilst such concentrating ability is retained in pre-renal AKI. The table below highlights important features that can be used to distinguish pre-renal AKI from ATN:

	Pre-renal	ATN
Urine osmolarity (mOsm/l)	> 500	< 350
Urine sodium (mmol/l)	< 20	> 40
Fractional sodium excretion	< 1%	> 2%
Urine/plasma urea	> 8	< 3
Urine/plasma creatinine	> 40	< 20

Longmore M, Wilkinson IB, Davidson EH et al. Oxford handbook of clinical medicine. Eighth edition. 2010.

15) E: Acute tubulo-interstitial nephritis

Although this patient developed an AKI nearly one week after a streptococcal sore throat, the development of arthralgia, fever, rash and an eosinophilia are collectively more in keeping with an acute interstitial nephritis. This is an immune-mediated hypersensitivity reaction, which most frequently occurs following exposure to certain drugs (usually antibiotics or NSAIDs) or following infections (e.g. staphylococcal, streptococcal). Renal biopsy findings typically reveal inflammatory cell infiltrates in the renal interstitium and tubules with T-cells and relative sparing of the glomeruli. Management relies on withdrawing the offending drug (if it's the precipitant) and a trial of steroids if appropriate.

Kodner CM and Kudrimoti A. Diagnosis and Management of Acute Interstitial Nephritis. American Academy of Family Physicians. 2003;67" 2527-34

16) E: Blocks the epithelial Na channel in the distal tubule and collecting ducts

Loop diuretics (e.g. furosemide and bumetanide) inhibit the Na-K-2Cl co-transporter in the thick ascending limb of the loop of henle.

Acetazolamide inhibits carbonic anhydrase.

Thiazide diuretics block the Na-Cl co-transporter in the distal tubules. Spironolactone is an example of an aldosterone receptor antagonist, whilst amiloride blocks amiloride-sensitive epithelial sodium channels in the distal tubules and collecting ducts.

17) D: Fluid challenge with 500ml gelofusine

This patient is septic. After securing the airway and giving oxygen, the next most important line of management is to gain intravenous access and give a fluid challenge since this patient is tachycardic and hypotensive. Giving a fluid challenge should have an almost immediate positive impact (unless the patient is truly shocked) and since this patient is haemodynamically compromised, it takes

A. Strongly negative birefringent needle-shaped crystals
B. Strongly negative birefringent rhomboid-shaped crystals
C. Weakly positive birefringent needle-shaped crystals
D. Weakly positive birefringent rhomboid-shaped crystals
E. Apple-green bi-refringence under polarised light

4) A 59-year old publican presents to his GP with an acutely painful left big toe. He is known to have gout, for which he is on allopurinol 300mg once a day.

The GP strongly suspects a diagnosis of an acute flare-up of gout.

Which of the following is the most appropriate line of management?

A. Stop allopurinol temporarily and start colchicine
B. Increase allopurinol to 600mg once daily
C. Stop allopurinol temporarily and start naproxen
D. Continue allopurinol and start naproxen
E. Continue allopurinol and start colchicine

5) All of the following drugs increases urate renal excretion EXCEPT:

A. Probenecid
B. Benzbromarone
C. Pyrazinamide
D. Sulfinpyrazone
E. High dose aspirin

6) A 76-year old lady presents with a 4-month history of progressive right anterior knee pain. The pain is exacerbated by long walks and climbing the stairs. She also complains of morning stiffness of her right knee, which often settles after 10 minutes.

Past medical history includes hypertension and angina.

She is currently taking paracetamol 1g four times a day for her knee pain.

On examination, she has a BMI of 32, there is limited active and passive range of movement of her right knee with evidence of crepitus.

An X-ray of her right knee shows some joint space narrowing with osteophytes.

Which of the following is the next step in management?

A. Celecoxib
B. Transcutaneous electrical nerve stimulation (TENS)
C. Oral NSAIDs
D. Topical NSAIDs
E. Surgical Arthroplasty

7) Your consultant asks you to review the radiograph of a hip. He explains that this patient is known to have osteoarthritis.

Which of the following is NOT a recognised radiographic sign of osteoarthritis?

A. Joint space narrowing
B. Osteophyte formation
C. Subchondral sclerosis
D. Subchondral bony cysts
E. Peri-articular osteopenia

8) A 67-year old man presents to his GP with a 4-month history of pain in his lower back and legs. Over the past month, he has noticed that he can no longer hear so well in his left ear.

On examination, the right tibia is bowed and is warm to touch.

Which of the following is most likely to be seen on a bone profile from this patient?

A. High Calcium, High Phosphate High ALP
B. High Calcium, Low Phosphate, High ALP
C. Normal Calcium, Normal Phosphate, Normal ALP
D. Normal Calcium, Normal Phosphate, High ALP
E. Normal Calcium, Low Phosphate, High ALP

9) A 73-year old woman presents to the rheumatology clinic with a 3-week history of morning stiffness, typically lasting an hour, and difficulty climbing the stairs. She complains of severe aching sensations of both her shoulders and hips, has become very lethargic and has lost 6 kg in weight over the last month.

She is mildly pyrexial with a temperature of 37.8 degrees.

Blood tests are as follows:

Hb	13.5	Na	136 mmol/l
MCV	89.0	K	4.3 mmol/l
Platelets	480	Creat	86 micromol/l
White cells	9.0	Urea	4.6 mmol/l
ESR	70 mm/hr	CRP	48

Which of the following is the most likely diagnosis?

A. Polymyalgia rheumatica
B. Polymyositis
C. Dermatomyositis
D. Fibromyalgia
E. Rheumatoid arthritis

10) A 76-year old female presents to her GP with a 1-week history of sudden onset right-sided headache. She complains of pain combing her hair and pain affecting her jaw muscles when chewing during meals. Yesterday, she experienced a transient episode of loss of vision

affecting her right eye, which appeared like a curtain descending over her vision.

Her past medical history includes polymyalgia rheumatica and hypothyroidism for which she takes levothyroxine replacement.

On examination, she has a thickened, tender right temporal artery.

Which of the following is the most appropriate treatment for this patient?

A. Oral prednisolone 10-20mg
B. Oral prednisolone 40-60mg
C. Intravenous hydrocortisone 100mg
D. Oral aspirin 300mg
E. Intravenous methylprednisolone 500mg-1g

11) A 54-year old lady presents to her GP with a 2-month history of painful and swollen fingers and wrists. There is no personal or family history of any dermatological condition.

On examination, most of the proximal interphalangeal (PIP) and metacarpophalangeal (MCP) joints bilaterally appear red, warm and tender to touch.

Investigations reveal:

Hb	10.8	Na	136 mmol/l
MCV	84.0	K	4.8 mmol/l
Platelets	584	Urea	3.2 mmol/l
White cells	9.4	Creat	102 micromol/l
Neutrophils	3.5		
CRP	84		
Rheumatoid factor	Negative		
Anti-CCP	Positive		

Which of the following is the most likely diagnosis?

A. Rheumatoid arthritis
B. Psoriatic arthritis
C. Reactive arthritis
D. Septic arthritis
E. Gout

12) Which of the following fulfils the diagnosis of Felty's syndrome:

A. Anaemia, hepatomegaly and rheumatoid arthritis
B. Anaemia, thrombocytopenia and rheumatoid arthritis
C. Thrombocytosis, anaemia and rheumatoid arthritis
D. Splenomegaly, neutropenia and rheumatoid arthritis
E. Rheumatoid arthritis and pneumoconiosis

13) Which of the following statements is FALSE regarding the management of rheumatoid arthritis (RA)?

A. Methotrexate, sulphasalazine and celecoxib have been shown to slow down the progression of the disease process and reduce joint destruction
B. Disease activity can be monitored using CRP and the DAS28 scoring system
C. A combination of DMARDs (methotrexate and at least one other DMARD) plus short-term glucocorticoids should be offered as first-line treatment
D. TNF-alpha inhibitors are indicated in patients that have failed to respond to a trial of at least 2 DMARDs
E. It often takes 6-12 weeks before symptomatic benefit is derived from DMARD therapy

14) A 23-year old student is reviewed by his GP. He complains of a 2-day history of increased redness, pain and swelling of his right knee joint. On further questioning, he suffered from a self-limiting diarrhoeal illness that lasted for 3 days nearly 2 weeks ago. He also complains of burning when passing urine and redness and soreness of both his eyes.

On examination, there is active inflammation of his right knee joint with range of movements significantly limited by pain. Visual fields and acuity are intact. Fundoscopy is unremarkable.

What is the most likely diagnosis?

A. Sjogrens Syndrome
B. Enteropathic arthritis
C. Reactive arthritis
D. Psoriatic arthritis
E. Still's disease

15) A 23-year old male student is reviewed by his GP. He complains of a 4-month history of lower back pain and stiffness. His symptoms are worse in the morning, usually lasting for at least 50 minutes to 1 hour, and are typically relieved by exercise.

On examination, there is no focal neurology, but reduced chest expansion and limited forward and lateral flexion of his lumbar spine.

What is the most likely diagnosis?

A. Mechanical back pain
B. Ankylosing spondylitis
C. Discitis
D. Slipped intervertebral disc
E. Spondylolisthesis

16) Which of the following is FALSE regarding seronegative spondyloarthropathies?

A. Patients are significantly more likely to be HLA-B27 positive compared with the general population
B. Rheumatoid factor is negative
C. Psoriatic arthritis is the commonest variant
D. Axial and polyarticular arthritis are not related to gastrointestinal disease activity in inflammatory bowel disease
E. Plantar fasciitis, Achilles tendonitis and costochondritis are well recognised clinical manifestations

17) Which of the following sequential colour changes characterises Raynaud's phenomenon?

    A. white → blue → red
    B. red→ blue → white
    C. white → red → blue
    D. red → white → blue
    E. blue → red → white

18) An elderly lady was recently diagnosed with limited cutaneous systemic sclerosis by her rheumatologist.

Which of the following antibodies is most closely associated with this condition?

    A. Anti-Scl70
    B. Anti-nuclear antibody
    C. Anti-histone antibody
    D. Anti-mitochondrial antibody
    E. Anti-centromere antibody

19) A 28-year old lady is reviewed in the rheumatology clinic. She presents with a 2-month history of pain and swelling of her fingers.

On examination, there is active inflammation predominantly affecting the distal interphalangeal (DIP) joints of both her hands, symmetrically. There is no evidence of skin lesions.

What is the most likely diagnosis?

    A. Rheumatoid arthritis
    B. Psoriatic arthritis
    C. Osteoarthritis
    D. Septic arthritis
    E. Reactive arthritis

20) A 43-year old male presents with a 4-month history of progressive, painless, proximal symmetrical muscle weakness.

On examination, there is a heliotrope discolouration around the eyelids, a violaceous papular eruption overlying the metacarpophalangeal (MCP) joints bilaterally and painful rough skin cracking over the tips and lateral aspects of most fingers.

Which of the following antibodies is most closely associated with this condition?

A. Anti-Ro
B. Anti-La
C. ANA
D. Anti-Sm
E. Anti-Mi-2

21) A 49-year old lady presents with a 6-month history of persistent dry eyes and dry mouth. Past medical history includes rheumatoid arthritis.

Which of the following tests can provide objective evidence of Sjogren's syndrome?

A. Schober's test
B. Pathergy test
C. Apley's test
D. Schirmer's test
E. Schilling's test

22) A 63-year old female presents with a 6-month history of a photosensitive facial rash, lethargy and arthralgia.

On examination, there is evidence of an erythematous rash on the face in a 'butterfly' pattern, with relative sparing of the nasolabial folds.

Observations are heart rate 78/min regular, blood pressure 148/84 mmHg and temperature 37.8 degrees.

Anti-histone antibodies are positive.

Which of the following is not a recognised cause for this condition?

A. Hydralazine
B. Pethidine
C. Procainamide
D. Isoniazid
E. Methyldopa

23) Which of the following is FALSE regarding systemic lupus erythematosus (SLE)?

A. Female to male ratio is approximately 9:1
B. It is more common in Afro-Carribeans than in Caucasians
C. Monthly intravenous "pulse" cyclophosphamide is a widely established treatment regimen in severe forms of lupus nephritis
D. Anti-smith antibodies are the most specific auto-antibodies for this condition
E. Patients with SLE tend to develop a destructive arthritis

24) Which of the following antibody-antigen associations is typical of Wegener's granulomatosis?

A. p-ANCA positive against MPO antigen
B. p-ANCA positive against PR3 antigen
C. c-ANCA positive against MPO antigen
D. c-ANCA positive against PR3 antigen
E. c-ANCA positive against RNP antigen

25) A 32-year old gentleman presents to the clinic with a 4-month history of lethargy, malaise and weight loss. Three weeks previously he has developed a left foot drop and persistent numbness affecting his right palm. He has also recently developed a painful ulcer on the dorsum of his right foot adjacent to his big toe.

On examination there is livedo reticularis, grade II weakness of left foot dorsiflexion and reduced sensation on his right hand in the median nerve distribution. A biopsy of the right foot ulcer is taken.

Investigations reveal:

FBC and U and Es normal
c-ANCA = negative
p-ANCA = negative
Normal C3/C4
Rheumatoid Factor - negative
Biopsy result = leukocytoclasis and fibrinoid necrosis in the medium sized-muscular arteries.

Which of the following viral infections is most strongly associated with this condition?

A. Epstein-Barr virus
B. Cytomegalovirus
C. Hepatitis B virus
D. Hepatitis C virus
E. HIV

Rheumatology Answers

1) B: Joint aspiration

The acutely hot and painful joint is a medical emergency. The first and foremost diagnosis that must be excluded is septic arthritis, as failure to promptly recognise and treat this condition can cause rapid irreversible joint destruction and in 11% of cases, mortality. The first-line investigation for an acute monoarthritis is joint aspiration.

The aspirate must be sent for microscopy, gram-staining, cultures and sensitivities. Blood cultures should be taken in anyone who is pyrexic on admission, but in the context of the acutely hot swollen joint, joint aspiration takes precedence. C-reactive protein (CRP) is non-specific and can be raised in virtually any infection or systemic inflammatory condition.

Plain radiographs of the affected joint are of no benefit in diagnosing or excluding septic arthritis, but can be useful in identifying chondrocalcinosis and chronic changes associated with certain arthritides (e.g. osteoarthritis). Arthroscopy is not a first-line investigation for the acutely inflamed joint but in the case of septic arthritis, can be used as a therapeutic method for cleaning and washing out the joint.

Other differential diagnoses for the acutely inflamed joint include gout, pseudogout, reactive, rheumatoid, psoriatic, enteropathic and osteo-arthritis.

BSR & BHPR, BOA, RCGP and BSAC guidelines for management of the hot swollen joint in adults. Rheumatology. 2006;45:1039-41

2) A: Staphylococcus aureus

Joint prostheses is one of several recognised risk factors for the development of septic arthritis; others being alcoholism, intravenous drug use, diabetes, previous intra-articular corticosteroid injections and cutaneous ulcers. Staphylococcus aureus is the most common cause of septic arthritis, closely followed by streptococci, which are both responsible for up to 91% of native joint infections. Septic arthritis can result from direct inoculation or more commonly, from haematogenous spread from another source of infection.

Although patients with prosthetic joint implants are at increased risk of infection by coagulase negative staphylococci, this predominantly applies to those with delayed presentations of septic arthritis (at least 3-months post-arthroplasty). Those presenting with early septic arthritis (within 3-months of arthroplasty) are most likely to culture Staphylococcus aureus similar to native joint infections.

Management of septic arthritis first requires resuscitation, joint aspiration (for diagnostic and therapeutic purposes), followed by commencement of intravenous antibiotics guided by local sensitivity patterns. IV antibiotics are often required for at least 2-weeks, followed by a minimum of 4-weeks oral antibiotics.

Urgent referral to an orthopaedic surgeon is essential in patients in whom the affected joint is prosthetic, so that prompt removal of the implant can be undertaken.

Brusch JL. Septic Arthritis. eMedicine. 2012.

Zimmerli W, Trampuz A, Ochsner PE. Prosthetic-joint infections. New England Journal of Medicine. *2004;351(16):1645-54*

Mathews CJ and Coakley G. Septic arthritis: current diagnostic and therapeutic algorithm. Current Opinion in Rheumatology. 2008; 20:457-62.

3) **A: Strongly negative birefringent needle-shaped crystals**

Affecting up to 1-2% of the adult population, gout is a prevalent inflammatory joint disease caused by the deposition of urate crystals in synovial joints. It classically affects the big toe (where it is referred to as podagra), but also commonly affects the foot, ankle, knee, wrists, fingers and elbows.

Joint aspirate findings under polarised light microscopy characteristically reveal the presence of strongly negative birefringent needle-shaped crystals; the colour of the crystals change from yellow to blue as the long-axis of the crystals rotates from a parallel to perpendicular orientation, compared with the plane of polarised light.

Weakly positive birefringent rhomboid-shaped crystals are typically found in pseudogout, an inflammatory arthropathy mediated by the deposition of calcium pyrophosphate crystals, more commonly affecting the knees and the older demographics than gout. Amyloid deposits in amyloidosis display apple-green birefringence under polarised light when stained with Congo red stain.

Underwood M. Diagnosis and management of gout. British Medical Journal. 2006;332:1315-19.

Jordan KM, Cameron S, Snaith M et al. British Society for Rheumatology and British Health Professionals in Rheumatology Guideline for the Management of Gout. Rheumatology. 2007; 46:1372-74

4) D: Continue allopurinol and start naproxen

Acute gouty flares are exquisitely painful and carry great morbidity. Affected joints should be rested and anti-inflammatories started promptly, usually for 1-2 weeks. Unless contraindicated, patients should receive short-term non-steroidal anti-inflammatory drugs (NSAIDs), like ibuprofen, diclofenac or naproxen. Patients at increased risk of peptic ulcers, GI bleeds or viscus perforations should be co-prescribed proton pump inhibitors (benefits versus risks of NSAIDs must be tailored according to each patient; if the risks of NSAIDs greatly outweigh the benefits, then alternative treatments must be considered). Second-line therapy for acute gout is colchicine, although its adverse effects (particularly diarrhoea) means that its use is not always very well tolerated by patients. Short-term steroid therapy is an effective alternative.

Allopurinol is a xanthine oxidase inhibitor and is used for gout prophylaxis. It should be considered in patients with recurrent attacks of gout (at least 2 attacks in one year) and in those with chronic tophaceous gout. Importantly, allopurinol must never be started for the first time during an acute flare of gout (as this can prolong the acute attack), but should be delayed by at least 1-2 weeks after the acute joint inflammation has settled. As highlighted by the BSR guidelines, patients already on allopurinol should continue it even during an acute attack of gout. Colchicine is a useful therapy for gout in the context of renal impairment.

Jordan KM, Cameron S, Snaith M et al. British Society for Rheumatology and British Health Professionals in Rheumatology Guideline for the Management of Gout. Rheumatology. 2007; 46:1372-74

5) C: Pyrazinamide

Anything that raises serum urate concentrations, whether it is by increasing urate production, or decreasing urate excretion, increases the risk of gout. Increased urate production can be secondary to a diet rich in purines (e.g. meat, fish, alcohol) or any condition associated with increased cell turnover such as lympho- or myeloproliferative disorders. Decreased urate excretion is most often due to drugs. For example, pyrazinamide, an anti-tuberculosis agent, and low dose aspirin, both reduce renal urate excretion. Note that although high serum urate concentrations are associated with an increased risk of gout, gout can still occur in patients with urate levels that lie within the normal range.

Underwood M. Diagnosis and management of gout. British Medical Journal. 2006;332:1315-19.

6) D: Topical NSAIDs

This patient has osteoarthritis (OA), which is the most common form of arthritis and a leading cause of morbidity worldwide. Pathophysiological changes underpinning OA include the localised loss of articular hyaline cartilage, joint space narrowing and bony remodelling with the formation of osteophytes.

OA is more common in women, older people, the obese, those with previous joint injuries and certain ethnic populations, with higher rates in Black and Chinese people than Caucasians. OA most commonly affects the knees, hips and small joints of the hand. Symptoms include pain, transient morning stiffness (less than 30 minutes) and reduced range of movement of the affected joint. Signs include crepitus, restricted movement and evidence of bony enlargement. Painless bony swellings can develop on the distal and proximal interphalangeal joints, where they are called Heberden's and Bouchard's nodes, respectively. In severe cases, patients may notice disabling catching/locking and sudden onset inability to fully extend the affected joint.

Management of OA should be conservative initially, encouraging weight loss, regular exercise and muscle strengthening exercises around the affected joint. NICE guidelines recommend the use of paracetamol as first-line analgesia, followed by topical NSAIDs, especially in those over 75 years of age. If these measures fail to control pain, then standard oral NSAIDs or certain COX-II selective inhibitors can be considered. NSAIDs should be avoided in those with previous peptic ulcers, heart failure and chronic kidney disease stage IV and V (with an eGFR<30ml/min).

When considering oral NSAIDs in those at increased risk of peptic ulceration, a proton pump inhibitor should also be prescribed. Opioids and intra-articular corticosteroid injections can be considered for analgesia, but should be reserved for second-line treatment if the aforementioned first-line treatments fail.

When OA becomes severely disabling and significantly impacts on patient quality of life, joint arthroplasty can be considered as a last resort, especially in cases of unremitting knee and hip OA.

National Institute for Health and Clinical Excellence. 2008. Osteoarthritis: The care and management of osteoarthritis in adults. CG59. London: National Institute for Health and Clinical Excellence.

Bennell KL, Hunter DJ and Hinman RS. Management of osteoarthritis of the knee. British Medical Journal. 2012; 345

7) E: Peri-articular osteopenia

Peri-articular osteopenia as well soft tissue swelling, bony erosions and joint space narrowing are all recognised radiological features of rheumatoid arthritis.

Fletcher DE and Rowley KA. The radiological features of rheumatoid arthritis. British Journal of Radiology. 1952; 25: 282-95

8) D: Normal Calcium, Normal Phosphate, High ALP

This patient is most likely to have Paget's disease of the bone. An understanding of the basic pathophysiological mechanisms underpinning this condition can make it easier to appreciate the symptoms and signs that can arise. In Paget's disease, osteoclasts are initially overactive, excessively lysing bone. Osteoblasts attempt to compensate by rapidly secreting large amounts of collagen, which comprise the osteoid bone matrix. Due to the high bone turnover, there is little time to organize the bone into regular lamellar arrangements. Therefore, the new bone is weak and patients are susceptible to pathological fractures, at the micro- and macroscopic level. This accounts for the bone pain. The synthesis of excess, disorganized bone by osteoblasts results in bony deformities, which can impinge on nerves. Most commonly cranial nerve VIII (vestibulocochlear) is compressed as it enters the internal acoustic meatus. This explains the sensorineural hearing loss.

The disorganized bone is highly vascular – warmth and in severe cases, high-output cardiac failure can result. Whenever there is a high turnover of cells, there is an increased risk for mutations to occur and therefore cancers to form. In this case, patients are at increased risk of osteosarcoma, which occurs in 1% of patients with Paget's disease.

Shaker JL. Paget's disease of bone: a review of epidemiology, pathophysiology and management. Therapeutic Advances in Musculoskeletal Disease. 2009;1:107-25

9) A: Polymyalgia rheumatica

This patient has polymyalgia rheumatica (PMR). It is a common condition, affecting women more than men (3:1 ratio), with an incidence of 100 per 100,000/year in those over 50, and almost never affects patients younger than this age. Characteristic clinical features include progressive proximal muscle pain, aches and stiffness, typically affecting the shoulder girdle muscles bilaterally, but often extending to affect the proximal hip muscles. Muscle strength is typically preserved. Proximal muscle stiffness is worse in the mornings and usually lasts for at least 45 minutes. Systemic symptoms include low-grade fever, depression and weight loss (but always inquire about features of potential underlying malignancy in any elderly patient presenting with weight loss!). Almost all patients with PMR have a raised ESR (usually over 50 mm/hr), often associated with a raised CRP. One of the most defining characteristics of PMR is a dramatic clinical response to low dose corticosteroids (10-20mg prednisolone in the morning) over 24-72 hours.

Polymyositis is a very rare inflammatory condition of the muscles with an estimated incidence of 0.5 per 100,000. Unlike PMR, polymyositis most often affects those between 45 and 54 years of age, is predominantly characterised by proximal muscle weakness, as opposed to stiffness (though pain and tenderness can occur), and can be associated with other symptoms such as dysphagia, arthritis and Raynaud's phenomenon. ESR can be raised in polymyositis, but an ESR above 50mm/hr is far more commonly seen in PMR. Creatine kinase is often elevated in polymyositis, but almost never raised in PMR. The management of polymositis also requires significantly higher doses of steroids (prednisolone 60mg/day or more) than PMR.

Patients with fibromyalgia often complain of chronic (> 3 months) generalised pain and widespread tenderness affecting at least 11 out of 18 designated tender points of the body. It is a non-inflammatory condition and a diagnosis of exclusion. Investigations are all normal and treatment includes reassurance, education, cognitive-behavioural therapy and long-term graded exercise programs. Patients rarely respond to steroids or non-steroidal anti-inflammatories.

Michet CJ and Matteson EL. Polymyalgia rheumatica. British Medical Journal. 2008; 336:765-69.

Hopkinson ND, Shawe DJ and Gumpel JM. Polymyositis, not polymyalgia rheumatica. Annals of the Rhematic Diseases. 1991;50:321-22.

10) E: Intravenous methylprednisolone 500mg-1g

This patient has giant cell arteritis (GCA), which is a common large vessel vasculitis. Patients are often elderly and can present with abrupt onset unilateral headache, scalp tenderness, jaw and tongue claudication, constitutional symptoms (e.g. fever, weight loss) and importantly, visual loss, which can affect up to 20% of patients. Patients with complicated GCA, that is the presence of jaw claudication or visual symptoms (amaurosis fugax in this case), must be treated with intravenous methylprednisolone 500mg-1g daily for 3 days followed by oral glucocorticoids, as they are at greatest risk of losing their sight. However, patients with uncomplicated GCA who lack such symptoms should be treated with 40-60mg oral prednisolone, which can be tapered down to a maintenance dose of 7.5-10mg once symptoms are controlled, for at least 2 years.

GCA is seen in approximately 30% of patients with polymyalgia rheumatica (PMR), so always inquire about headache and the aforementioned symptoms in patients with suspected PMR. ESR is often elevated in GCA, but the gold-standard diagnostic investigation is temporal artery biopsy. Skip lesions can produce false-negative results, so samples should be at least 1cm in length.

Dasgupta B, Borg FA, Hassan N et al. BSR and BHPR guidelines for the management of giant cell arteritis. Rheumatology. 2012;49:1594-7

11) A: Rheumatoid arthritis

Rheumatoid arthritis (RA) is a chronic, autoimmune, inflammatory and often symmetrical polyarthritis, with a predilection for the small joints. It most commonly affects PIPs, MCPs, metatarsophalangeal (MTP), wrist and ankle joints, but can also involve the knees, hips, shoulders and elbows. Its prevalence is 1%, it is twice as common in women than men and its incidence peaks in the 5th to 6th decade of life.

Rheumatoid factor is an auto-antibody present in 70% of patients with RA, therefore a negative rheumatoid factor does not exclude the diagnosis. However, it's not very specific as it can be positive in conditions including systemic sclerosis, autoimmune hepatitis, subacute bacterial endocarditis, systemic lupus erythematosus and primary biliary cirrhosis amongst others. Anti-cyclic citrullinated peptide (anti-CCP) antibodies are more specific than rheumatoid factor for RA.

The diagnostic criteria for RA are shown below:

At least 4 of the following should be present. Numbers 1-4 should be of at least 6 weeks' duration:

1) *Morning stiffness for > 1 hour*
2) *Synovitis in 3 or more joints*
3) *Synovitis in the hands or wrists*
4) *Symmetrical distribution*
5) *Subcutaneous nodules*
6) *Positive rheumatoid factor*
7) *Radiographic changes on X-rays of the hands or wrists*

New classification criteria for RA have been developed:

Joint involvement* (0-5)	Score
1 medium-large joint	**0**
2-10 medium-large joints	**1**
1-3 small joints (with or without involvement of large joints)	**2**
4-10 small joints (with or without involvement of large joints)	**3**
>10 joints (at least one small joint)	**5**

Serology	
Negative rheumatoid factor and negative anti-CCP antibodies	**0**
Low positive rheumatoid factor or low positive anti-CCP antibodies	**2**

High positive rheumatoid factor or high positive **3**
anti-CCP antibodies

Acute phase reactants
Normal CRP and normal ESR   **0**
Abnormal CRP or abnormal ESR   **1**

Duration of symptoms
<6 weeks   **0**
>6 weeks   **1**

*Large joints refers to shoulders, elbows, hips, knees and ankles
*Small joints refers to MCP, PIPs, 2ⁿᵈ to 5ᵗʰ MTPs, thumb IP joints and wrists

A score of at least 6/10 points is needed for a definite diagnosis of RA. Patients with RA who are positive for rheumatoid factor are more likely to follow an aggressive disease course with extra-articular manifestations, which include:

1) Skin – rheumatoid nodules (most common; 30% of patients)
2) Pulmonary – exudative pleural effusions, diffuse interstitial fibrosis, bronchiolitis obliterans
3) Vasculitis (can cause mononeuritis multiplex due to inflammation of the vasa nervorum, and thus neurological symptoms)
4) Cardiac – ischaemic heart disease, pericarditis (rarely symptomatic), myocarditis
5) Renal - glomerulonephritis
6) Haematological – anaemia, thrombocytopenia/thrombocytosis, neutropenia
7) Ocular – keratoconjunctivitis sicca (at least 10% of patients), episcleritis, scleritis
8) Gastrointestinal – GI problems most likely iatrogenic, e.g. secondary to NSAIDs, but very rarely intestinal infarction can occur as a result of mesenteric vasculitis

In the rheumatology OSCE, you may be faced with a patient with advanced clinical features of RA and be asked to examine their hands, of which the following findings are classical:

a) A symmetrical, deforming polyarthropathy typically affecting the MCPs and PIPs. If the joints are red, swollen, tender and warm to touch, then there is active synovitis.

b) Radial deviation at the wrists with ulnar deviation at the MCPs

c) Subluxation of the proximal phalanges at the MCPs

d) Boutonniere deformity of the fingers; fixed flexion deformity at the PIP and hyperextension at the distal interphalangeal (DIP) joints of the same finger.

e) Swan neck deformity; hyperextension at the PIP and fixed flexion at the corresponding DIP joints

f) Z-thumb

g) Wasting of the instrinsic hand muscles secondary to disuse, and thenar muscle wasting, which could be secondary to median nerve compression (RA patients are at increased risk of carpal tunnel syndrome).

Aletaha D, Neogi T, Silman AJ et al. 2010 Rheumatoid Arthritis Classification Criteria; An American College of Rheumatology/ European League Against Rheumatism Collaborative Initiative. Arthritis & Rheumatism. 2010;62: 2569-81

Klarenbeek NB, Kerstens P JSM, Huizinga T WJ, Dijkmans B AC and Allaart C F. Recent advances in the management of rheumatoid arthritis. British Medical Journal. 2011;342:39-44

Young A. Koduri G. Extra-articular manifestations and complications of rheumatoid arthritis. Best Practise & Research Clinical Rheumatology. 2007;21:907-27

12) D: Splenomegaly, neutropenia and rheumatoid arthritis

Felty's syndrome is a triad of rheumatoid arthritis, splenomegaly and neutropenia. The combination of rheumatoid arthritis and pneumoconiosis secondary to exposure to coal dust, asbestos or silica, is called Caplan's syndrome.

13) A: Methotrexate, sulphasalazine and celecoxib have been shown to slow down the progression of the disease process and reduce joint destruction

DMARDs (Disease Modifying Anti-rheumatic Drugs) include methotrexate, sulphasalazine, hydroxychloroquine, leflunomide and gold. Patients that have failed to respond to at least 2 DMARDs qualify for a trial of TNF-alpha inhibitors, examples being adalimumab, etarnecept and infliximab.

DMARDs have been proven to slow down the pathophysiological progression of the disease process underpinning rheumatoid arthritis.

They can slow down structural damage of affected joints and improve long-term prognosis, especially if utilised early in the disease. NSAIDs and COX-II inhibitors (e.g. celecoxib), however, purely provide symptomatic relief and have no impact on halting disease progression.

National Institute for Health and Clinical Excellence. 2007. Adalimumab, etanercept and infliximab for the treatment of rheumatoid arthritis. CG130. London: National Institute for Health and Clinical Excellence.

National Institute for Health and Clinical Excellence. 2009. The management of rheumatoid arthritis. CG79. London: National Institute for Health and Clinical Excellence.

Deighton C, O'Mahony R, Tosh J, Turner C and Rudolf M. Management of rheumatoid arthritis: summary of NICE guidance. British Medical Journal. 2009;338:b702

Emery P. Treatment of rheumatoid arthritis. British Medical Journal. 2006;332:152-5

14) C: Reactive arthritis

This patient presents with an acute inflammatory mono-arthritis, urethritis and conjunctivitis. The triad is called Reiter's syndrome, which represents a subset of reactive arthritis (not all patients with reactive arthritis develop this triad of symptoms). Reactive arthritis is a mono- or oligoarthritis classically occurring 1-3 weeks post-urogenital infection (typically caused by ureaplasma urealyticum or chlamydia trachomatis) or post-dysenteric infection (typically Campylobacter, Salmonella, Yersinia or Shigella). The arthritis is usually a mono- or oligoarthropathy affecting the lower limb joints. Not all patients with reactive arthritis have urethritis or conjunctivitis. Management includes resting the affected joints, NSAIDs and/or local steroid injections.

Although septic arthritis is less likely than reactive arthritis given the history, the inflamed joint must still be aspirated in order to exclude this possibility. Importantly, an aspirate of the inflamed joint in a patient with reactive arthritis is *sterile*.

Wu IB, Schwartz RA. Reiter's syndrome: the classic triad and more. Journal of the American Academy of Dermatology. *2008;59:113-21.*

Carter JD, Hudson AP. Reactive arthritis: clinical aspects and medical management. Rheumatic Diseases Clinics of North America. *2009;35:21-44*

15) B: Ankylosing spondylitis

Ankylosing spondylitis (AS) is one of several seronegative spondyloarthropathies. It is more common in men (5:1 male to female ratio) and peak age of onset is 15-35 years. It is characterised by inflammation of the sacroiliac joints (sacroiliitis), spine and the entheses (i.e. points of attachment between tendon, capsule or ligaments to bone). As the inflammatory process progresses, bony syndesmophytes form, which bridge the vertebrae and induce spinal ankylosis (i.e. the vertebrae become locked in position). In advanced disease, patients develop the characteristic 'question mark posture.'

Making the diagnosis requires the presence of low back pain for at least 3 months (often associated with stiffness, worse in the mornings lasting for at least 45 minutes and relieved by exercise), limitation of lumbar spinal flexion in the frontal and sagittal planes and/or decreased chest expansion. First-line investigation is with an X-ray of the sacro-iliac joints in order to detect radiographic evidence of sacroiliitis.

Management is conservative and includes encouraging exercise (not rest!), physiotherapy and NSAIDs for pain relief. The TNF-alpha inhibitors adalimumab, etanercept and more recently golimumab have recently been recommended by NICE in a certain subset of AS patients.

McVeigh CM and Cairns AP. Diagnosis and management of ankylosing spondylitis. British Medical Journal. 2006;333: 581-85

National Institute for Health and Clinical Excellence. 2008. Adalimumab, etanercept and infliximab for ankylosing spondylitis. CG143. London: National Institute for Health and Clinical Excellence.

National Institute for Health and Clinical Excellence. 2011. Golimumab for the treatment of ankylosing spondylitis. CG233. London: National Institute for Health and Clinical Excellence.

16) C: Psoriatic arthritis is the commonest variant

The seronegative spondyloarthropathies represent a group of inflammatory arthritides that share common clinical and aetiological features as shown below:

1) HLA-B27 association (only 5% in the general population, but found in up to 90% of certain types of seronegative spondyloarthritis)
2) Seronegativity – rheumatoid factor negative
3) Axial arthritis – with inflammation affecting the sacro-iliac joints and/or spine
4) Asymmetrical oligoarthritis with fewer than 5 large joints being affected or a symmetrical small-joint polyarthritis, which can mimic rheumatoid arthritis
5) Dactylitis – inflammation of entire digits
6) Enthesitis –examples include plantar fasciitis, costochondritis and Achilles tendonitis.
7) Extra-articular manifestations – anterior uveitis, apthous oral ulcers, psoriaform rashes, aortic valvular incompetence

The different types of seronegative spondyloarthropathies are:

Ankylosing spondylitis (AS) – This is the commonest variant. Up to 90% of patients are HLA-B27 positive.

Psoriatic arthritis – associated with psoriasis. However, the occurrence of arthritis can precede, by up to a number of years, the formation of a rash. Different variants exist, which are discussed later.

Enteropathic arthritis – This is arthritis associated with inflammatory bowel disease (IBD). It is the commonest extra-intestinal manifestation, affecting up to 30% of patients with IBD (commoner in crohn's disease). Three different variants exist: axial arthritis, oligoarthritis and polyarticular arthritis. Axial arthritis affects the sacroiliac joints or spine producing features similar to AS.

Oligoarthritis affects fewer than 5 large joints such as the hips, knees, ankles, wrists, elbows and shoulders. It is usually asymmetric, acute and self-limiting. Polyarticular arthritis affects 5 or more joints, often symmetrically, usually the small joints of the hand. Unlike asymmetrical oligoarthritis, axial and polyarticular arthritis are both unrelated to gastrointestinal disease activity.

Reactive arthritis – An aseptic mono or oligoarthritis, which occurs 1-3 weeks post-urogenital or gastrointestinal infection.

Undifferentiated spondyloarthritis – has clinical features of seronegative spondyloarthritis, which don't quite fit into the 4 aforementioned categories.

Longmore M, Wilkinson I, Davidson E, Foulkes A and Mafi A. Oxford Handbook of Clinical Medicine. Eighth Edition.

Zochling J and Smith EUR. Seronegative spondyloarthritis. Best Practise & Research Clinical Rheumatology. 2010;24:747-56.

Larsen, S., Bendtzen, K. and Neilsen, O.H. Extraintestinal manifestations of inflammatory bowel disease: epidemiology, diagnosis, and management. Annals of Medicine 2010; 42: 97-114.

17) A: white → blue → red

Raynaud's phenomenon is characterised by typical sequential colour changes in the digits owing to vasospasm (classically from white to blue to red). Sudden constriction of digital vessels limits blood flow to the digits, causing pallor (white). Prolonged constriction results in a peripheral cyanosis as the local concentration of deoxy-haemoglobin rises in the digital vessels. Sudden dilatation of the digital vessels leads to a reactive hyperaemia accounting for the final red colour change, which may be associated with pain and throbbing. Occasionally the colour can change straight from pallor to red if vasoconstriction is not sufficiently prolonged.

Primary Raynaud's phenomenon (Raynaud's disease) is idiopathic and comprises up to 90% of cases. Secondary Raynaud's phenomenon is more severe, associated with complications (e.g. digital ulcers) and is due to an underlying cause, such as connective tissue disorders spanning systemic sclerosis, systemic lupus erythematosus, rheumatoid arthritis, Sjogren's, polymyositis and dermatomyositis. Primary and secondary Raynaud's can be differentiated on the basis of capillaroscopy. Management includes conservative measures by encouraging patients to wear gloves to keep their hands warm, avoid cold and to try calcium channel blockers and angiotensin II receptor blockers. In refractory cases, prostaglandin analogues and endothelin receptor antagonists may trialled. Addressing Secondary Raynaud's will also require treatment of the underlying condition.

Levien TL. Advances in the treatment of Raynaud's phenomenon. Vascular Health and Risk Management. 2010;6:167-77

18) E: Anti-centromere antibody

Systemic sclerosis is characterised by the deposition of abnormally high amounts of collagen from overactive fibroblasts, leading to fibrosis of subcutaneous and cutaneous tissues and in severe cases, internal organs. Skin thickening, hardening and tightening due to skin sclerosis gives rise to characteristic clinical manifestations. These include microstomia with accompanying radial furrowing around the mouth, 'beak nose' deformity and sclerodactyly. Raynaud's phenomenon is ubiquitous in systemic sclerosis. Prolonged ischaemia to the digits can cause painful ulceration, nail dystrophy and even amputation.

Two main forms of systemic sclerosis exist, which are limited and diffuse cutaneous systemic sclerosis:

1) <u>Limited cutaneous systemic sclerosis (lcSSC)</u> – skin sclerosis is limited to the peripheries distal to the knees and elbows. Pulmonary fibrosis and isolated pulmonary hypertension are recognised associations (though pulmonary fibrosis is more commonly seen in the diffuse form). A subset of lcSSC is called CREST – a syndrome encompassing a constellation of Calcinosis, Raynaud's phenomenon, (o)Esophageal dysmotility, Sclerodactyly and Telangiectasia. The presence of anti-centromere antibody is one of the hallmarks of this condition.

2) <u>Diffuse cutaneous systemic sclerosis (dcSSc)</u> – This heralds a poorer prognosis. More extensive skin sclerosis extending to proximal to the elbows and knees, and even affecting the trunk occurs in the diffuse variant. Internal organ involvement is more frequently seen, which can cause pulmonary fibrosis and hypertensive renal crises. Antibodies associated with dcSSc include anti-topisomerase 1 (also called anti-Scl 70) and anti-RNA polymerases I and III antibodies, the latter conferring an increased risk of renal involvement. Management often requires steroids and strong immunosuppressants.

Derret-Smith EC and Denton CP. Systemic sclerosis: clinical features and management. Medicine. 2009;38: 109-15

19) B: Psoriatic arthritis

The prevalence of inflammatory arthritis in the general population is approximately 2-3%, but in patients with psoriasis, the prevalence is 6-42%. The absence of psoriasis does not exclude a diagnosis of psoriatic arthritis, however, as the development of the rash may occur for up to several years after the joints have been affected. Rheumatoid arthritis tends to spare the DIPs.

Different clinical patterns of joint involvement in psoriatic arthritis have been recognised including:

1) Asymmetric oligoarthritis (<5 joints),
2) Symmetric polyarthritis, predominantly affecting the MCPs and PIPs (mimicking rheumatoid arthritis)
3) Distal arthritis (predominantly affecting the DIPs as in this patient)
4) Spondyloarthritis (sacroiliitis and spondylitis)
5) Arthritis mutilans

Gladman DD, Antoni C, Mease P, Clegg DO and Nash P. Psoriatic arthritis: epidemiology, clinical features, course, and outcome. Annals of the Rheumatic Diseases. 2005;64:ii14-ii17

Scottish Intercollegiate Guidelines Network. Diagnosis and management of psoriasis and psoriatic arthritis in adults. Guideline 121. 2010.

20) E: Anti-Mi-2

This patient has dermatomyositis. This is characterised by a relatively painless progressive proximal muscle weakness (like polymyositis) along with fairly classical dermatological manifestations spanning Gottron's papules (the rash over the knuckles, which can also be present over PIPs and DIPs), the heliotrope rash and 'mechanics hands' (the painful skin cracking).

Antibody associations are commonly asked about in examinations as they represent a frequent pitfall.

The following are classical antibody-disease associations in rheumatology:

1) Rheumatoid factor – rheumatoid arthritis (70%), Sjogren's disease, autoimmune hepatitis, infective endocarditis.
2) Anti-CCP – more specific antibody for rheumatoid arthritis
3) ANA (anti-nuclear antibody) – systemic lupus erythematosus (SLE), Sjogren's, autoimmune hepatitis

4) Anti-smooth muscle antibody – autoimmune hepatitis, SLE
5) Anti-double stranded DNA antibodies – more specific antibody for SLE than ANA (anti-Smith being most specific for SLE)
6) Anti-Ro (SSA) – SLE, Sjogren's, systemic sclerosis; transplacental passage of this antibody to the fetus can cause congenital conduction heart block
7) Ant-La (SSB) – Sjogrens, SLE
8) Anti Jo-1 and anti-Mi-2 – polymyositis and dermatomyositis
9) Anti-histone – drug-induced lupus

Dalakas MC and Hohlfeld. Polymyositis and dermatomyositis. The Lancet. 2003;362: 971-82

21) D: Schirmer's test

Sjogren's syndrome is a chronic autoimmune disorder associated with the destruction of the exocrine glands. It can occur alone (primary Sjogren's) or in conjunction with an underlying autoimmune disorder such as rheumatoid arthritis, systemic sclerosis or systemic lupus erythematosus (secondary Sjogren's).

Patients have dry eyes (keratoconjunctivitis sicca) and mouths (xerostomia) for at least 3 months.

Objective evidence of dry eyes can be provided by employing Schirmer's test, which involves placing paper strips onto the lower eyelids for 5 minutes to measure tear production. The test is positive if less than 5 mm of the paper strip is moistened over 5 minutes.

Schober's test is used to check the degree of lumbar flexion. A mark is placed at around the level of the Dimples of Venus, and 1 finger 5cm below and a second finger 10cm above this mark. If the increase in distance between the 2 fingers is less than 5 cm as the patient tries to touch their toes with their legs straight, then the test is positive signifying limited lumbar flexion suggestive of ankylosing spondylitis.

Pathergy is a test for Behcet's disease. Schilling's and Mantoux tests are used in suspected pernicious anaemia and TB screening, respectively.

Fox RI. Sjogren's syndrome. Lancet. 2005;366:321-31

22) B: Pethidine

This patient has drug-induced lupus. More than 95% of patients with this condition test positive for anti-histone antibodies. Drugs most strongly associated with this condition include hydralazine, procainamide, isoniazid, methyldopa, quinidine, minocycline and chlorpromazine.

Vasoo S. Drug-induced lupus: an update. Lupus. 2006;15:757-61

23) E: Patients with SLE tend to develop a destructive arthritis

SLE is a multisystem autoimmune connective tissue disorder with a diverse array of clinical presentations. It is far commoner in females (9:1 female to male ratio) and commoner amongst certain ethnicities, such as people with African or Asian ancestry.

The diagnostic criteria for SLE are shown below (adapted from the 1982 revised criteria for the classification of SLE):

1) *Malar rash* – fixed erythema, flat or raised, over the malar eminences, tending to spare the nasolabial folds (the classical 'butterfly' facial rash)
2) *Discoid rash* – erythematous raised patches with adherent keratotic scaling and follicular plugging; atrophic scarring may occur in older lesions
3) *Photosensitivity* – skin rash provoked or exacerbated by sunlight
4) *Oral ulcers* – oral or nasopharyngeal ulceration, which are often painless
5) *Arthritis* – a non-erosive arthritis characterised by tenderness, swelling or effusion; a reversible deforming arthropathy can result, which is called *'Jaccoud's arthropathy.'*
6) *Serositis* – pleuritis or pericarditis

7) *Renal* – may manifest as the nephritic or nephrotic syndrome. Renal manifestations are not always symptomatic.

8) *Neurological* – seizures or psychosis (although 19 different CNS syndromes are now recognised)

9) *Haematological disorders* – haemolytic anaemia, leucopenia, lymphopenia and/or thrombocytopenia can result

10) *Immunological findings* – including anti-double stranded DNA, anti-Smith or anti-phospholipid antibody

11) Abnormally high titre of *antinuclear antibody*

A diagnosis of SLE is made if at least 4 out of the 11 criteria are met at any point in time. As well as pericarditis, cardiac involvement includes Libman-Sacks endocarditis and accelerated rates of ischaemic heart disease (as with all chronic inflammatory conditions).

Hydroxychloroquine is the mainstay for treating patients with mild lupus and in maintenance therapy, often in association with NSAIDs for symptomatic relief. Low dose steroids may also be used in maintenance, but their side effects limit their use. Steroid sparing agents such as azathioprine, methotrexate and mycophenolate mofetil are very useful treatments.

Acute severe flare-ups of lupus (e.g. in lupus nephritis, severe pericarditis or CNS disease) require intravenous cyclophosphamide and high dose steroids.

D'Cruz DP. Systemic lupus erythematosus. British Medical Journal. 2006; 332:890-4

Tan EM, Cohen AS, Fries JF. The 1982 revised criteria for the classification of systemic lupus erythematosus. Arthritis and rheumatism. 1982;25: 1271-77.

24) D: c-ANCA positive against PR3 antigen

ANCA stands for anti-neutrophil cytoplasmic antibodies, which are positive in certain types of vasculitides.

p-ANCA and c-ANCA are distinct antibodies that differ in their staining patterns; they follow a peri-nuclear and cytoplasmic staining pattern, respectively.

c-ANCA antibodies are most commonly found in Wegener's granulomatosis whereas p-ANCA antibodies are less specific, being frequent in microscopic polyangiitis, Churg-Strauss syndrome and ulcerative colitis.

c-ANCA and p-ANCA antibodies target PR3 and MPO antigens, respectively.

25) C: Hepatitis B virus

This patient has polyarteritis nodosa (PAN), a rare necrotising vasculitis with a striking predilection for the medium-sized muscular arteries. It spares the aorta and its major branches, and spares the capillaries, small arterioles that lack muscular coats and the venous system.

Clinical manifestations include constitutional symptoms common to many conditions such as fever, lethargy, malaise, myalgia, anorexia and weight loss. More specific presenting features include:

1) Mononeuritis multiplex – damage to 2 or more peripheral nerves, in the case of vasculitides like PAN, is secondary to inflammation of the vasa nervorum.
2) Cutaneous features – livedo reticularis, nodules, ulcerations and digital ischaemia
3) Renal – microaneurysms in the kidneys, intraparenchymal renal inflammation, renal infarcts. PAN does not cause glomerulonephritis.
4) Gastrointestinal – mesenteric ischaemia causing 'post-prandial angina,' and rarely in more severe cases acute bowel infarction.
5) Genitourinary – orchitis and ovarian inflammation

Cardiac lesions are mostly subclinical in PAN.

Clinical features that separate PAN from other ANCA-associated vasculitides, namely wegener's granulomatosis and microscopic polyangiitis include the absence of glomerulonephritis and the sparing of lung involvement in PAN, as well as the differing patterns of serology (PAN is usually negative for ANCA).

Of the mentioned viruses, PAN is most strongly associated with hepatitis B, with up to 30% of patients being infected.

Essential mixed cryoglobulinaemia, strongly associated with viral hepatitis C, is commonly accompanied by a low C4 and a strongly positive rheumatoid factor.

Stone JH. Polyarteritis nodosa. JAMA. 2002; 288:1632-9

Haematology Questions

1) Which of the following is TRUE regarding the mutation that forms haemoglobin S?

   A. Substitution: valine is replaced by glutamate in the beta globin chain
   B. Substitution: glutamate is replaced by valine in the alpha globin chain
   C. Substitution: glutamate is replaced by valine in the beta globin chain
   D. Production of fewer alpha globin chains
   E. Production of fewer beta globin chains

2) A 23-year old Afro-Carribean male presents to the emergency department with a 2-hour history of very severe, sudden onset lower back pain and pain in the right lower leg. He denies any other symptoms.

   The patient is known to have sickle cell disease and recognises this type of pain as a typical painful sickle cell crisis.

   Which of the following represents the most appropriate first-line analgesic in the acute setting for this patient?

   A. Intravenous paracetamol
   B. Intramuscular pethidine
   C. Intramuscular diclofenac
   D. Oral morphine
   E. Intravenous morphine

3) You are asked to review a 28-year old African lady, known to have sickle cell disease.

   She was originally admitted due to an acute painful sickle cell crisis, and despite remaining on 10 days of patient-controlled analgesia (PCA), she complains of ongoing pain affecting her left leg.

   On examination, there is warmth, redness, swelling and tenderness over the left tibia.

Observations are heart rate 118/min regular, blood pressure 110/82mmHg and temperature 37.8 degrees at present. You note that the patient has been spiking temperatures of over 38 degrees during the last few days.

Bloods reveal rising inflammatory markers with a most recent CRP of 320. X-ray left tibia shows evidence of osteomyelitis.

Which of the following is the most likely causative organism given this clinical picture?

A. Eschericia coli
B. Staphyloccocus aureus
C. Salmonella typhimurium
D. Haemophilus influenza
E. Enterobacter species

4) Which of the following is NOT a recognised feature of haemolytic anaemia?

A. Raised serum LDH
B. Raised serum haptoglobin
C. Haemoglobinuria
D. Indirect hyperbilirubinaemia
E. Reticulocytosis

5) A 42-year old lady presents with a 1-week history of progressive dyspnoea and malaise.

The patient was diagnosed with systemic lupus erythematosus (SLE) 2 years ago.

She is markedly pale on examination. Investigations reveal:

Hb	8.2 g/dl
MCV	102 fl
Reticulocyte count	6% (normal range 0.5-1.5%)
Direct Coombs test	Positive

Peripheral blood smear shows multiple erythrocytes with reduced central pallor.

Which of the following is the MOST likely diagnosis?

A. Cold autoimmune haemolytic anaemia
B. Warm autoimmune haemolytic anaemia
C. Microangiopathic haemolytic anaemia
D. Alloimmune haemolytic anaemia
E. Hereditary spherocytosis

6) An 18-year old female student presents with a 5-day history of severe lethargy, fatigue, sore throat and loss of appetite.

On examination there is tender anterior and posterior cervical lymphadenopathy and exudative pharyngitis with bilateral tonsillar enlargement.

The patient is pyrexic with a temperature of 38.2 degrees.

Investigations show:

FBC:	Normocytic anaemia with an Hb of 8.4g/dl
Direct Coombs' test	Positive
Cold agglutinins	Positive
Monospot test	Positive

What is the most likely cause of this clinical presentation?

A. Cytomegalovirus (CMV)
B. Parvovirus B-19
C. Streptococcus
D. Toxoplasmosis
E. Epstein-Barr Virus (EBV)

7) A 28-year old teacher presents with a 5-day history of lethargy and malaise superimposed on a 1-week history of cough and coryzal symptoms.

On examination, he is jaundiced and there is mild splenomegaly. Peripheral blood smear shows spherocytes. Osmotic fragility test is positive.

Which of the following is the most common mode of inheritance of this condition?

A. Autosomal dominant
B. Autosomal recessive
C. X-linked recessive
D. X-linked dominant
E. Co-dominant

8) A 35-year old lady of Middle Eastern origin presents with a 48-hour history of severe abdominal pain, shortness of breath and lethargy.

On examination, there is conjunctival pallor and icterus.

Blood film shows evidence of Heinz Bodies and bite cells.

Which of the following is the most likely diagnosis?

A. Acute intermittent porphyria
B. Hereditary spherocytosis
C. Haemolytic uraemic syndrome
D. Favism
E. Autoimmune haemolytic anaemia

9) A 30-year old lady originally from South East Asia is brought to the emergency department with a 3-day history of severely progressive fatigue, generalised weakness and pallor.

Bloods reveal a profound drop in haemoglobin from her normal baseline of around 7.5 g/dl to an Hb of 3.2 g/dl.

Which of the following is the most likely cause?

A. Cytomegalovirus (CMV)
B. Parvovirus B-19
C. Epstein-Barr virus (EBV)
D. Toxoplasmosis
E. Human Immunodeficiency virus (HIV)

10) Which of the following statements regarding thalassaemias are INCORRECT?

A. Beta thalassaemias arise due to mutations of beta globin genes on chromosome 11
B. Haemoglobin H disease occurs secondary to dysfunction of 3 alpha globin genes
C. Haemoglobin Bart's predominates in cases of hydrops foetalis
D. Skull X-rays in patients with thalassaemia major characteristically show the pepper pot sign
E. Target cells and poikilocytes are found in peripheral blood smears

11) A 42-year old gentleman presents to the emergency department with a 3-day history of acute confusion, severe lethargy and general deterioration.

On examination, there is a widespread petechial rash, jaundice and pyrexia of 38.4 degrees.

Bloods reveal:

Hb	7.2	(11-14)	Na	136	(135-145)
MCV	84.0	(84-99)	K	4.2	(3.5-4.5)
Platelets	62	(150-400)	Creat	384	(baseline 110)

Peripheral blood smear – evidence of schistocytes

What is the most appropriate first line management?

A. Platelet transfusion
B. Combined red cell and platelet transfusion
C. High dose steroids
D. Intravenous cyclophosphamide
E. Plasma exchange

12) A 73-year old gentleman is seen in the outpatient clinic. He presents with a 3-month history of PR bleeding and weight loss.

A full blood count reveals an Hb of 9.2g/dl.

Which of the following is INCORRECT concerning this type of anaemia?

A. It is associated with microcytosis
B. Serum ferritin is typically reduced
C. Serum soluble transferrin receptors usually raised
D. Serum iron is reduced
E. Serum total iron binding capacity is reduced

13) Which of the following regarding the storage of blood products is CORRECT?

A. Red cells are stored at 4°C and have a shelf life of up to 15 days
B. Red cells are stored at 4°C and have a shelf life of up to 25 days
C. Platelets are stored at 22°C on an agitator and have a shelf life of 8 days
D. Fresh frozen plasma is stored at -30°C and has a shelf life of up to 12 months
E. Fresh frozen plasma is stored at -30°C and has a shelf life of up to 24 months

14) A 33-year old male who was admitted to hospital due to an upper GI bleed secondary to duodenal ulceration is due to receive 2 units of red cells.

Approximately 10 minutes into receiving the transfusion, he becomes flushed, anxious and develops sudden onset back pain.

On examination, the patient looks generally unwell, has rigors and a temperature of 38.6 degrees.

What is the most likely diagnosis?

A. Acute febrile non-haemolytic transfusion reaction
B. ABO incompatible haemolytic transfusion reaction
C. Transfusion associated graft-versus-host disease (TA-GvHD)
D. Anaphylaxis
E. Transfusion-related acute-lung injury (TRALI)

15) A 29-year old lady who is 33 weeks pregnant presents to the emergency department with sudden onset lower abdominal pain and vaginal bleeding.

No foetal heart sounds are audible.

Observations are heart rate 86/min and regular, blood pressure 126/82 mmHg, temperature 36.9 degrees and oxygen saturations 96% on air.

Bloods reveal:

Hb	9.2 g/dl	(11-14)
Platelets	80 x 10^9/l	(150-400)
PT	19 secs	(11-15 secs)
aPTT	49 secs	(35-45 secs)
Fibrinogen	0.8	(1.5 -3g/l)

Which of the following is the first most appropriate line of management?

A. 2 units cross matched red cells
B. FFP
C. Platelets
D. Cryoprecipitate
E. Prothrombin complex concentrate

16) A 64-year old man presents to his GP with a 6-week history of fatigue and new onset upper back pain. There is no significant past medical history.

On examination, there is midline tenderness over T6. Investigations show:

Hb	9.6 g/dl
MCV	85
Platelets	340
ESR	84 mm/hr

Serum electrophoresis = positive for monoclonal paraprotein
Urine Bence-Jones protein = positive

What is the most likely diagnosis?

A. Monoclonal gammopathy of undetermined significance (MGUS)
B. Myelodysplasia
C. Myelofibrosis
D. Multiple myeloma
E. Osteoporotic wedge fracture

17) A 68-year old man presents to the assessment unit with a 1-day history of increasing confusion and drowsiness after a fall.

CT head shows a large subdural haematoma.

He is on warfarin for atrial fibrillation.

His INR is 10.

What is the most appropriate management?

A. Stop warfarin and give oral vitamin K
B. Omit warfarin dose for 2 days, then recheck INR
C. Stop warfarin and give intravenous vitamin K
D. Stop warfarin and give intravenous vitamin K and dried prothrombin complex concentrate
E. Stop warfarin and give intravenous vitamin K and FFP

18) Which of the following combination of clotting factors does warfarin interfere with the synthesis and function of?

A. II, VIII, IX, X
B. II, VII, IX, X
C. II, VIII, X, XI
D. II, VII, X, XI
E. VII, IX, X, XI

19) Which of the following clotting results are characteristic of haemophilia A?

(aPTT = activated partial thromboplastin time, PT = prothrombin time, TT= thrombin time)

A. Prolonged aPTT, normal PT, normal TT
B. Prolonged aPTT, prolonged PT, prolonged TT, prolonged reptilase time
C. Prolonged aPTT, prolonged PT, prolonged TT, normal reptilase time
D. Normal aPTT, normal PT, prolonged TT
E. Normal aPTT, prolonged PT, normal TT

20) Which of the following is NOT a recognised cause of massive splenomegaly?

A. Chronic Myeloid Leukaemia (CML)
B. Visceral Leishmaniasis
C. Myelofibrosis
D. Malaria
E. Chronic Lymphocytic Leukaemia

21) A 68-year old male is referred to the haematology clinic. He originally presented with a 5-month history of malaise, weight loss and abdominal discomfort.

Bloods show a marked leukocytosis with basophilia, eosinophilia and thrombocytosis. Philadelphia chromosome is positive.

Which of the following is the first line treatment?

A. Imatinib
B. Interferon alpha
C. Steroids
D. Thalidomide
E. Vincristine

22) A 24-year old female was recently diagnosed with acute myeloid leukaemia M3.

What is the most appropriate treatment combination?

A. ATRA and arsenic trioxide
B. ATRA and arsenic dioxide
C. ATRA and arsenic monoxide
D. Cyclophosphamide
E. Interferon and dexamethasone

23) Which of the following chromosomal translocations is most frequently seen in Burkitt's lymphoma?

A. t(9;22)
B. t(8;14)
C. t(15;17)
D. t(14;18)
E. t(11;14)

24) A 58-year old Caucasian male is reviewed in clinic.

He originally presented with a 4-month history of lassitude, frequent headaches, dizziness and visual disturbances. He also reports symptoms consistent with erythromelalgia and pruritis exacerbated by warm baths.

On examination, he has a plethoric complexion and is hypertensive.

Mutations in which of the following genes, is most commonly found in the primary form of this disorder?

A. cMYC
B. nMYC
C. JAK-2
D. PRV
E. TEL

25) A 33-year old female presents with an 8-week history of intermittent fever, weight loss and drenching night sweats.

On examination, there is painless rubbery inguinal lymphadenopathy.

A CT chest-abdo-pelvis also reveals enlarged mediastinal lymph nodes. The bone marrow and liver are not involved.

An excisional lymph node biopsy of the affected inguinal nodes is performed, which shows Reed Sternberg cells.

A diagnosis of Hodgkin's lymphoma is made.

What stage does this patient fall in to?

A. Stage Ia
B. Stage IIa
C. Stage IIb
D. Stage IIIa
E. Stage IIIb

26) A routine blood test carried out on a patient in a GP surgery shows:

Hb	10.2	(11-14)
MCV	112	(84-99)
Platelets	460	(150-400)
White cells	9.2	(3.7-8.7)

Which of the following is LEAST likely to cause the above blood results?

A. B12 deficiency
B. Folate deficiency
C. Hypothyroidism
D. Haemolytic anaemia
E. Iron deficiency

Haematology Answers

1) C: Substitution: glutamate is replaced by valine in the beta globin chain

Sickle cell disease is an autosomal recessive disorder that represents a major cause of morbidity worldwide. Patients with sickle cell anaemia are homozygous for the haemoglobin S mutation (HbS). HbS results from a substitution mutation whereby glutamic acid in position 6 of the beta globin chain is replaced by valine. In the deoxygenated form, HbS forms polymers, which disrupts the architecture and flexibility of the erythrocyte, resulting in the characteristic sickle cell shape.

A distinction must be made between sickle cell disease and sickle cell anaemia. Sickle cell anaemia is the most common form of sickle cell disease. Patients with sickle cell anaemia are homozygous for the HbS mutation and suffer from one of the most severe clinical phenotypes. Patients whom are compound heterozygotes for HbS carry the HbS gene and another abnormal haemoglobin gene (e.g. HbC). Compound heterozygotes generally have a less severe clinical phenotype than homozygotes for HbS. Patients who carry the HbS gene along with a normal adult haemoglobin gene (HbA) are said to have sickle cell trait and because they very rarely suffer from complications, they are not considered to have sickle cell disease.

Rees DC, Williams TN and Gladwin MT. Sickle-cell disease. Lancet. 2010;376:2018-31

Steinberg MH. Sickle Cell Anemia, the First Molecular Disease: Overview of Molecular Etiology, Pathophysiology, and Therapeutic Approaches. TheScientificWorldJOURNAL. 2008. 8:1295-1324.

2) E: Intravenous morphine

The clinical manifestations of sickle cell disease arise from two key pathophysiological processes: acute vaso-occlusive crises and haemolytic anaemia. Severe acute vaso-occlusive episodes predominantly account for the occurrence of acute sickle cell crises. The sickle shaped erythrocytes can occlude the microvasculature and cause local tissue ischaemia and infarction.

The most obvious symptom of sickle cell crisis is pain, which is frequently excruciating in acute crises (often disproportionate to examination findings). Patients can complain of severe chest pain, back pain, abdominal pain (which may mimic an acute abdomen) and/or pain in the limbs.

Treatment of sickle cell crises include:

a) Oxygen – not routinely given unless the patient is hypoxic
b) Effective analgesia - In adults, first-line analgesia in the acute setting should be in the form of parenteral opiates (either IV or subcutaneous), preferably morphine or diamorphine. Pethidine is not recommended. Mild or moderate background pain may be controlled with paracetamol and nonsteroidal anti-inflammatory drugs (NSAIDs), progressing to stronger analgesics if pain remains uncontrolled. In children, severe painful crises can be managed with strong oral opiates first-line.
c) IV fluids
d) Broad spectrum antibiotics – this is indicated in patients if they have chest symptoms (e.g. in acute chest syndrome, see later) or if an underlying infection is suspected. Ideally, blood cultures should be taken before antibiotics are given.
e) Thromboprophylaxis – sickle cell crises represent a prothrombotic state and patients must be started on low molecular weight heparin and given TEDS stockings unless contraindicated.
f) Blood transfusion or exchange transfusion – these patients are typically transfused if their haemoglobin drops below 5g/dl. Severe chest crises, suspected cerebrovascular events or multi-organ failure merit exchange transfusion, whereby blood is removed from the patient and replaced with transfused blood.

Management of chronic disease involves:

a) *Hydroxycarbamide* – if patients suffer frequent crises. This works by increasing HbF (foetal haemoglobin) synthesis and reducing the degree of sickling.
b) *Managing hyposplenism* – repeated splenic infarcts can cause functional hyposplenism. Such patients should be appropriately immunised (standard immunisation schedule, plus annual

influenza and five-yearly pneumococcal vaccine) and be given prophylactic antibiotics.

c) *Bone marrow transplant* – this is the only possible curative option but remains controversial.

Rees DC, Olujohungbe AD, Parker NE, Stephens AD, Telfer P and Wright J. Guidelines for the management of the acute painful crisis in sickle cell disease. British Journal of Haematology. *2003;120:744-52*

3) C: Salmonella typhimurium

Patients with sickle cell disease are susceptible to a myriad of complications, of which osteomyelitis is one example, as in this case.

Many of these complications can arise as a result of vaso-occlusive episodes, the consequences of which vary according to the location of the microvasculature affected.

Vaso-occlusion in the:

a) Lungs – can cause acute chest syndrome due to acute lung infarction, inflammation and infection. Patients can develop dyspnoea, tachypnoea, chest pain, fever and cough. New pulmonary infiltrates are seen on chest radiography. In severe circumstances, patients can develop acute respiratory distress syndrome. Chronic vaso-occlusion can lead to pulmonary hypertension.

b) Brain – vaso-occlusion can cause cerebrovascular events. Up to 11% of patients have had a stroke by 20 years of age. Ischaemic strokes are commoner in children, whereas haemorrhagic strokes are more likely in adults, secondary to rupture of aneurysms (probably the result of persistent vascular injury).

c) Spleen – vaso-occlusion can lead to cumulative splenic infarction leading to hyposplenism. This is a major cause of immunodeficiency in sickle cell patients, rendering them at significantly increased risk of infection by encapsulated bacteria (i.e. Pneumococcus, Meningococcus and Haemophilus Influenza type B). Patients with such functional hyposplenism, or who have had a splenectomy, should be offered penicillin prophylaxis.

d) Kidneys – renal infarction can cause papillary necrosis and renal failure.

e) Bone – occlusion of the bone medullary vessels can lead to avascular necrosis. Infarcted bone is at increased risk of infection, causing osteomyelitis. For reasons that are unclear, osteomyelitis in sickle cell patients is most likely to be caused by Salmonella infection as opposed to Staphylococcus Aureus, which is the commonest cause in the general population.

f) Urogenital – priapism is a urological emergency which, unless treated promptly, can cause impotence and further morbidity.

Almeida A and Roberts I. Bone involvement in sickle cell disease. British Journal of Haematology. 2005;129;482-90.

4) B: Raised serum haptoglobin

Haemolytic anaemia produces a stereotypical pattern of laboratory test results summarised below:

a) *Anaemia* – reduced haemoglobin, which is most often normocytic, but can be macrocytic

b) *Reticulocytosis* – the bone marrow attempts to compensate for the loss of red cells by increasing the rate of erythropoiesis. This ultimately manifests in the blood as an increase in the reticulocyte count (reticulocytosis), which represent the immediate precursors to erythrocytes. As reticulocytes are larger than red cells, with an average MCV of 150fl, haemolytic anaemia can be associated with a macrocytosis.

c) *Raised serum lactate dehydrogenase (LDH)* – LDH is an enzyme found in high concentrations within red cells, and is consequently released into the plasma following haemolysis.

d) *Haemoglobinaemia, haemoglobinuria and reduced haptoglobin* haemolysed cells directly release haemoglobin into the circulation causing haemoglobinaemia. Haptoglobin, a protein predominantly synthesised by the liver, binds free circulating haemoglobin, the complexes then being cleared by the reticuloendothelial system. If the rate of haemolysis is particularly high and haptoglobin levels are rapidly depleted, excess haemoglobin becomes filtered by the kidneys and appears in the urine (haemoglobinuria) causing it to be dark, or even black.

e) *Unconjugated hyperbilirubinaemia* – excess haem metabolism in the liver increases the production of unconjugated bilirubin (also known as indirect bilirubin), causing affected patients to appear jaundiced. Patients with chronic haemolytic anaemia are at increased risk of gallstones (of the pigment variety) and corresponding pathological sequalae including biliary colic, acute cholecystitis, pancreatitis and cholangitis.

Haemolytic anaemia can be divided into hereditary and acquired forms:

Hereditary haemolytic anaemia

a) Membranopathies, e.g. hereditary spherocytosis
b) Enzymopathies, e.g. G6PD deficiency
c) Haemoglobinopathies, e.g. sickle cell disease, thalassaemias

Acquired haemolytic anaemia

a) Immune-mediated, e.g. autoimmune, alloimmune, drug-induced
b) Microangiopathic haemolytic anaemia, e.g. thrombotic thrombocytopenic purpura (TTP), haemolytic uraemic syndrome (HUS), disseminated intravascular coagulation (DIC), prosthetic valves, pre-eclampsia, malignant hypertension
c) Infection, e.g. malaria

Dhaliwal G, Cornett PA and Tierney LM. Hemolytic Anemia. American Family Physician. 2004;69: 2599-606.

5) B: Warm autoimmune haemolytic anaemia

This patient presents with a 1-week history of symptomatic anaemia. The macrocytosis is a consequence of the reticulocytosis. The Direct Coombs' test, also known as the direct antiglobulin test, is used to demonstrate the presence of antibodies or complement proteins bound to antigens on the surface of the red blood cells. If the red cells agglutinate in the presence of specific anti-human immunoglobulins, then the test result is positive. A positive Direct Coombs' test is highly suggestive of autoimmune haemolytic anaemia (AIHA). AIHA can be divided into warm and cold subtypes, and each can be further subdivided into primary (idiopathic) or secondary (where there is an underlying cause). These are discussed further below:

Warm AIHA

a) It's driven by autoantibodies that undergo maximal antigen binding at a temperature of 37 degrees
b) Accounts for 48-70% of AIHA
c) Principally IgG-mediated
d) Most common secondary causes include lymphoproliferative disorders like chronic lymphocytic leukaemia (CLL), Hodgkin's and non-Hodgkin's lymphoma, and Waldenstrom's macroglobulinaemia. Other secondary causes include autoimmune disorders such as SLE, rheumatoid arthritis and scleroderma.

Cold AIHA

a) Driven by autoantibodies that undergo optimal binding at colder temperatures (0-4 degrees).
b) Less common than warm AIHA
c) Principal8ly IgM-mediated
d) Secondary causes are predominantly lymphoproliferative disorders (CLL, lymphoma, Waldenstrom's macroglobulinaemia) and infections, typically infectious mononucleosis and Mycoplasma pneumonia.

Autoimmune disorders are more strongly linked with warm AIHA. The past medical history of SLE thus makes warm AIHA the most likely diagnosis. Note that the formation of spherocytes occurs in both hereditary spherocytosis and AIHA. They appear in AIHA because as the antibody-coated cells enter the spleen, parts of the red cell membrane become phagocytosed, reducing the surface area, which transforms the biconcave shape to a sphere.

*Gehrs BC and Friedberg RC. Autoimmune Hemolytic Anemia.
American Journal of Haematology. 2002;69:258-71*

6) E: Epstein-Barr Virus (EBV)

The diagnosis is infectious mononucleosis (also called glandular
fever), which is caused by infection with the Epstein-Barr Virus
(EBV). The Monospot test detects heterophile antibodies frequently
found in patients with infectious mononucleosis. Although the test
carries a high specificity, false positives can occur in leukaemia,
CMV, toxoplasmosis and parvovirus B-19 infection. However,
the occurrence of cold autoimmune haemolytic anaemia clinches
the diagnosis, as it is most strongly associated with infectious
mononucleosis from the options listed.

The Monospot and Paul-Bunnell tests, which are employed to aid in
the diagnosis of this condition, involve mixing the patients serum
with horse or sheep red cells, respectively. The tests are positive when
red cell agglutination occurs due to the interaction with heterophile
antibodies in the serums of infected patients.

Although the clinical picture of infectious mononucleosis can
resemble streptococcal sore throat, it is imperative not to treat
patients suffering from infectious mononucleosis with penicillin as
this can notoriously cause a severe rash.

*Luzuriaga K and Sullivan JL. Infectious Mononucleosis. The New
England Journal of Medicine. 2010; 362:1993-2000*

7) A: Autosomal dominant

This patient has hereditary spherocytosis (HS), which is the most
common inherited anaemia in the Northern European population,
affecting up to 1 in 2000 people. 75% of cases are inherited in
an autosomal dominant manner, the remainder being autosomal
recessive. The pathophysiology of HS lies in a defect in one of several
proteins that constitute part of the membranous skeleton required
for maintaining the integrity and shape of red cells, whilst ensuring
their deformability as they enter the microcirculation. Red cells in

HS patients are more fragile and vulnerable to haemolysis. Genetic defects have been identified in several different proteins including ankyrin, alpha and beta spectrin, band 3 and protein 4.2.

Spherocytes in HS have a shorter lifespan reduced from the normal 120 days of biconcave healthy erythrocytes, to only a few days. Whilst patients are commonly asymptomatic, episodes of haemolytic anaemia can be provoked, most often by intercurrent illness or infection.

One of the key management decisions for HS, which also applies to other haemolytic anaemias, is when to pursue splenectomy. As most spherocytes are destroyed by the spleen, splenectomy will help to significantly reduce the likelihood of haemolytic episodes. However, splenectomised patients are rendered highly vulnerable to potentially severe and overwhelming sepsis. All splenectomised patients are at increased risk of infection by encapsulated bacteria, which include pneumococcus, meningococcus and haemophilus influenza type B. Thus, all patients should be offered vaccination against these bacteria before splenectomy and lifelong penicillin prophylaxis after splenectomy to reduce the risk of sepsis.

Perrotta S, Gallagher PG and Mohandas N. Hereditary spherocytosis. Lancet. 2008;372: 1411-26.

Bolton-Maggs PHB. Hereditary spherocytosis; new guidelines. Archives of Disease in Childhood. 2004;89: 809-12

8)   D: Favism

This patient has glucose-6-phosphate dehydrogenase (G6PD) deficiency, the most common enzymopathy (inherited in an X-linked recessive pattern) causing haemolysis. The highest prevalence is found in the Middle East, tropical Africa, certain parts of Asia and the Mediterranean.

G6PD is an enzyme that catalyses the first reaction in the pentose phosphate pathway and is essential for the production of reduced NADP (i.e. NADPH), which subsequently reduces the oxidised form of the tri-peptide, glutathione. Reduced glutathione is needed for lowering the levels of oxidative stress in cells. Patients with G6PD deficiency are highly susceptible to haemolytic anaemia induced by oxidative damage, when exposed to certain insults that increase levels of oxidative stress. Under such toxic circumstances, the haemoglobin undergoes denaturation and forms small inclusion bodies within the erythrocytes called Heinz bodies; these are subsequently removed by the spleen leaving remnants of erythrocytes that appear as if part of them have been bitten away, hence the term bite cells (also known as degmacytes). Note that Heinz bodies are not pathognomonic for G6PD deficiency as they can also be seen in certain conditions like chronic liver disease.

Haemolytic episodes in G6PD deficiency typically occur 2 to 4 days following infection, exposure to certain drugs or foods (classically fava beans, causing favism). Drugs commonly implicated in inducing haemolytic anaemia in G6PD deficiency include primaquine, dapsone, nitrofurantoin to name but a few.

Mehta A, Mason PJ and Vulliamy TJ. Glucose-6-phosphate dehydrogenase deficiency. Bailliere's Clinical Haematology. 2000; 13: 21-38.

9) B: Parvovirus B-19

This patient who has low baseline haemoglobin, which could be secondary to iron-deficiency anaemia or thalassaemia, presents with aplastic crisis exemplified by the precipitous drop in haemoglobin.

The most common aetiology for aplastic crisis is parvovirus B-19 infection, which targets the erythroprogenitor cells in the bone marrow causing temporary red cell aplasia. An acute aplastic crisis only occurs in patients who have an already reduced red cell lifespan, such as those with iron deficiency anaemia, thalassaemia, sickle cell disease or hereditary spherocytosis. In healthy individuals, parvovirus B-19 is often asymptomatic or manifests as a self-limiting non-specific flu-like illness – aplastic crisis doesn't result because the normal erythrocyte lifespan of 120 days is long enough to mask the effects of transient red cell aplasia.

Servey JT, Reamy BV and Hodge J. Clinical Presentations of Parvovirus B19 infection. American Family Physician. 2007;75:373-6

10) D: Skull X-rays in patients with thalassaemia major characteristically show the pepper pot sign

The 'hair-on-end' appearance is usually seen in thalassaemia major and represents extramedullary haematopoiesis. The pepper pot sign is a sign of multiple myeloma.

Thalassaemias represent one of the hereditary haemoglobinopathies characterised by a reduced or absent synthesis of globin chains. In alpha and beta thalaessaemia, there is a reduced synthesis of alpha and beta globin chains, respectively.

Alpha thalassaemia

There are normally two active alpha globin genes on each copy of chromosome 16. Alpha thalassaemia arises as a consequence of deletion of 1 or more alpha globin genes:

a) *Deletion of 1 alpha gene* (α^+ thalassaemia heterozygous; $\alpha,-/\alpha,\alpha$) patients are asymptomatic but routine laboratory testing reveal borderline Hb and MCV with low MCH.

b) *Deletion of 2 alpha genes* (α^+ thalassaemia homozygous; $\alpha,-/\alpha,-$ or α^0 thalassaemia heterozygous; α,α /-,-) – patients are asymptomatic but laboratory testing reveals slight anaemia with low MCV and MCH

c) *Deletion of 3 alpha genes* (Haemoglobin H disease; $\alpha,-/-,-$) – patients are anaemic with very low MCV and MCH. Clinical features of chronic haemolytic anaemia arise including hepatosplenomegaly, gallstones, jaundice and leg ulcers. Other problems include skeletal changes such as prominent frontal bossing (due to ineffective erythropoiesis causing extramedullary bone marrow expansion), osteopenia and pathological fractures. Patients may need blood transfusions if significant haemoglobin drops occur e.g. secondary to aplastic crisis.

d) *Deletion of 4 alpha genes* (Hydrops foetalis; -,-/-,-) – foetal haemoglobin ($\alpha 2/\gamma 2$) cannot be produced, meaning that haemoglobin Bart's ($\gamma 4$), which is non-functional, predominates. Death commonly occurs in utero secondary to severe anaemia and heart failure.

Beta thalassaemia

There is normally one active beta globin gene on each copy of chromosome 11. Beta thalassaemia arises as a consequence of mutations, more than 200 of which have been identified (spanning deletions and substitutions), in one or both of these beta globin genes. The classification of beta thalassaemia is shown below:

a) *Beta Thalassaemia major* (deletion of both beta globin genes) – Clinical features of haemolytic anaemia develop from around 3 months of age when the levels of foetal haemoglobin normally drop. Patients develop feeding problems, growth retardation, poor muscular development as well as significant hepatosplenomegaly, pathological fractures and skeletal defects secondary to extramedullary bone marrow expansion (similar to haemoglobin H disease). The latter accounts for frontal bossing and maxillary hyperplasia ('thalassaemic facies'). Typical skull X-ray findings are the 'hair-on-end' appearance. Unless proper treatment is instituted, life expectancy is 5-10 years. Patients require life-long regular blood transfusions to maintain haemoglobin above 9.5 g/dl. Complications of iron-overload from chronic transfusion should be monitored and prevented using iron chelators (e.g. desferrioxamine parenteral infusions).

b) *Beta Thalassaemia intermedia* (many different genotypic combinations exist) – patients are anaemic with very low MCV and MCH, but symptoms are less profound and have a later onset than thalassaemia major as some beta globin synthesis is preserved. Patients typically maintain a haemoglobin of more than 7g/dl and have variable transfusion dependency.

c) *Beta Thalassaemia trait* (deletion of one beta globin chain) – patients are clinically asymptomatic with routine laboratory tests showing slight anaemia with low MCV and MCH. A diagnosis is most often made by identifying an HbA2 ($\alpha 2\delta 2$) of more than 4% using high performance liquid chromatography (HPLC), normal values being below 3.5%.

HPLC, like capillary electrophoresis, can be employed to separate out the different haemoglobin components seen in both normal and diseased states, such as HbA (normal; α2β2.), HbF (foetal; α2γ2), HbA2 (α2δ2), HbH (β4) and Hb Barts (γ4).

Peters M, Heijboer H, Smiers F and Giordano PC. Diagnosis and management of thalassaemia. British Medical Journal. 2012;344:e228

11) E: Plasma exchange

This patient has Thrombotic Thrombocytopenic Purpura (TTP), one of many causes of microangiopathic haemolytic anaemia (i.e. anaemia resulting from shearing of red cells as they pass through fibrin-impregnated turbulent microcirculations). It is a rare haematological emergency characterised by a pentad of symptoms and signs:

a) Neurological disturbance (e.g. confusion, seizures, coma, focal neurological deficits, which may be transient)
b) Fever
c) Microangiopathic haemolytic anaemia
d) Thrombocytopenia
e) Acute kidney injury

Under normal circumstances, monomers or small multimers of von Willebrand Factor (vWF), which are responsible for driving platelet aggregation, are derived from the cleavage of larger multimers of vWF by the enzyme ADAMTS-13 (a disintegrin and metalloproteinase with thrombospondin-1-like domains). In TTP, ADAMTS-13 activity is profoundly reduced (usually to 0-5% of normal activity) resulting in the persistence of these unusually large vWF multimers in the circulation, which are pathologically more effective in inducing platelet aggregation. Widespread platelet aggregation, particularly concentrated within the cerebral and renal circulations, ultimately cause the symptoms and signs seen in TTP. As the red cells flow through the affected platelet and fibrin-occluded microvasculature, they are physically sheared and torn apart, causing schistocytosis and intravascular haemolytic anaemia.

In reality, many patients with TTP do not present with the whole pentad of symptoms and signs. Indeed, many patients solely present with evidence of thrombocytopenia and microangiopathic haemolytic anaemia. Although rare, TTP carries a very high mortality unless managed promptly. Treatment of choice is plasma exchange.

Haemolytic-uraemic syndrome (HUS), another thrombotic microangiopathy, presents as acute kidney injury and microangiopathic haemolytic anaemia. Although there is much overlap between the clinical features of TTP and HUS, there are certain differentiating factors. Patients with HUS tend to have greater renal involvement, they often present about a week after a diarrhoeal illness (typically caused by E. coli 0157:H7 or Shigella Dysenteriae) and have preserved ADAMTS-13 activity.

Other causes for microangiopathic haemolytic anaemia include malignant hypertension, disseminated intravascular coagulation (DIC), prosthetic heart valves and obstetric disorders like pre-eclampsia.

Moake JL. Thrombotic Microangiopathies. The New England Journal of Medicine. 2002;347: 589-600.

Allford SL, Hunt BJ, Rose P, Machin SJ; Haemostasis and Thrombosis Task Force, British Committee for Standards in Haematology. British Journal of Haematology. 2003;120: 556-73

12) E: Serum total iron binding capacity is reduced

This patient has iron deficiency anaemia (IDA), which represents the most common cause of anaemia worldwide. The commonest cause of IDA in men and postmenopausal women is blood loss from the gastrointestinal tract. In this scenario, given the patient's old age, history of weight loss and PR bleeding, colorectal malignancy must be excluded.

IDA is associated with microcytosis and a reduced serum iron and ferritin, whilst serum soluble transferrin receptors and total iron binding capacity are usually elevated. Note that a normal ferritin does not exclude iron deficiency, as it is an acute phase reactant that can be raised to within the normal range in iron deficient patients if there is an on-going inflammatory process. Additionally, if iron and B12/folate deficiency co-exist, the microcytosis (caused by iron deficiency) and macrocytosis (caused by B12 and/or folate deficiency) may essentially average out and produce a normocytic picture.

Liu K and Kaffes AJ. Iron deficiency anaemia: a review of diagnosis, investigation and management. European journal of gastroenterology & hepatology. 2012;24: 109-16

13) E: Fresh frozen plasma is stored at -30°C and has a shelf life of up to 24 months

Red cells are stored at 4°C and have a shelf life of up to 35 days.

Platelets are stored on a platelet agitator close to room temperature at 22°C and have a shelf life of 5 days.

Fresh frozen plasma is stored at -30°C and has a shelf life of up to 24 months.

McClelland DBL (Editor). Handbook of Transfusion Medicine. United Kingdom Blood Services 4th Edition. 2007.

14) B: ABO incompatible haemolytic transfusion reaction

Infusion of ABO incompatible blood is most commonly due to clerical errors and represents the most frequent cause of adverse transfusion events. This error may occur in taking or labelling the sample, collecting the wrong blood from the fridge, or failure to undertake the required checks immediately before transfusion has started.

The following outlines the recognised complications that can occur as a result of blood transfusion:

Acute complications

a) *ABO incompatible haemolytic transfusion reaction* – an easily avoidable life threatening adverse reaction. Anti A and/or anti B antibodies from the patient react with A and/or B antigens in the donor blood leading to severe haemolysis, activation of the complement system and disseminated intravascular coagulation. Symptoms shortly develop even after a few mls of incompatible blood has been transfused. Patients rapidly deteriorate and become generally unwell, develop chills, fever, chest/back/abdominal pains and shock.

b) *Acute febrile non-haemolytic transfusion reaction* – affects 1-2% of recipients and clinical features include fever (>1.5°C above baseline), often accompanied by shivering and generalised discomfort. This reaction is not life-threatening but it's important to note that fever may be the first sign of a more severe acute reaction (such as ABO incompatibility)

c) *Anaphylaxis* – a life-threatening allergic reaction. Patients develop bronchospasm, urticaria, erythema and periorbital and laryngeal oedema. Shock rapidly ensues.

d) *Bacterial infection* – patients can develop fever, rigors and shock. Bacterial contamination of blood products is more often associated with platelet transfusions (as platelets are stored at 22 °C) than with red cells (stored at 4 °C).

e) *Transfusion-related acute lung injury (TRALI)* – Occurs within six hours of transfusion. Patients develop acute respiratory distress syndrome characterised by non-cardiogenic pulmonary oedema manifesting as tachypnoea, non-productive cough, hypoxia and bilateral pulmonary infiltrates on chest x-ray. The pathogenesis is thought to arise secondary to antibodies in the donor plasma interacting with the recipient's neutrophils.

f) *Transfusion-associated circulatory overload (TACO)* – excessive and rapid blood transfusions in susceptible patients (e.g. those with poor LV function and elderly frail patients) can lead to acute left ventricular failure. This can be avoided by administering 20-40mg furosemide with each or alternative units of blood depending on the clinical situation.

Delayed complications

a) *Delayed haemolytic transfusion reaction* – occurs more than 24 hours after transfusion. Features include fever and symptoms and signs of haemolysis. Antibodies against Kidd and Rhesus systems are the most frequent cause.

b) *Tranfusion associated graft-versus-host disease (Ta-GvHD)* – engraftment and proliferation of transfused lymphocytes from the donor in susceptible recipients (immunocompromised patients) can result in fever, skin rash, hepatitis and diarrhoea. It has a high mortality and outlines the need to transfuse immunocompromised patients at risk with irradiated blood products to inactivate donor lymphocytes and reduce the risk of this condition.

c) *Post-transfusion purpura* – the development of anti-platelet antibodies in the recipient can cause severe thrombocytopenia. It occurs 5-9 days post-transfusion.

d) *Secondary haemochromatosis* – patients who receive regular life-long blood transfusions (e.g. those with thalassaemia) are at risk of developing iron overload; this risk is reduced through the use of iron chelating agents such as desferrioxamine.

PHB Bolton-Maggs (Ed) and H Cohen on behalf of the Serious Hazards of Transfusion (SHOT) Steering Group. The 2011 Annual SHOT Report (2012)

McClelland DBL (Editor). Handbook of Transfusion Medicine. United Kingdom Blood Services 4th Edition. 2007.

15) D: Cryoprecipitate

This woman presents with placental abruption, which has been complicated by disseminated intravascular coagulation (DIC). DIC is characterised by a delocalised, systemic activation of pathways leading to and regulating the coagulation system. This leads to the disseminated formation of microthrombi throughout the systemic vasculature, which can cause multi-organ failure owing to disrupted organ perfusion. The deposition of fibrin throughout the microvasculature haemolyses red cells and results in micro-angiopathic haemolytic anaemia with schistocytosis. Rapid consumption of clotting factors and platelets simultaneously leads to an increased risk of bleeding. Thus DIC is a paradoxical clinical state encompassing concurrent thrombosis and haemorrhage, ultimately heralding a poor prognosis with high morbidity and mortality.

Patients with DIC and bleeding, or at high risk of bleeding, should be offered platelet transfusion if the platelet count is less than 50 x 10^9/l. Prophylactic platelet transfusion in non-bleeding patients is generally offered at a higher threshold of 10-20 x 10^9/l, although management must be tailored according to clinical need. A haemoglobin of less than 8 is generally considered the threshold for transfusion of red cells, explaining why option A is incorrect.

The prothrombin time (PT) and activated partial thromboplastin time (aPTT) are prolonged in around 50-60% of patients with DIC at some point during their illness, so normal clotting times does not exclude a diagnosis of DIC. Although this patient has mildly prolonged clotting times, it is the severe hypofibrinogenaemia (defined as <1g/l) that needs to be corrected first. This is best achieved with cryoprecipitate.

The following conditions are associated with DIC:
Sepsis and severe infection
Pancreatitis
Trauma
Malignancy
   -Solid tumours or leukaemia, especially acute pro-myelocytic leukaemia

Obstetric
   -Placental abruption
   -Pre-eclampsia
   -Amniotic fluid embolism

Severe liver failure
ABO transfusion incompatibility
Transplant rejections

It is important to note that the management of DIC should ultimately be based on treating the underlying condition and taking the clinical state of the patient into central consideration. It should not solely be based on correcting the various laboratory parameters.

Levi M and Ten Cate H. Disseminated intravascular coagulation. The New England Journal of Medicine. 1999;341:586-92

Levi M, Toh CH, Thachil J and Watson HG. Guidelines for the diagnosis and management of disseminated intravascular coagulation. British Committee for Standards in Haematology. British Journal of Haematology. 2009;145:24-33.

16) D: Multiple myeloma

Multiple myeloma accounts for 10% of all haematological malignancies and is caused by the malignant clonal proliferation of plasma cells in the marrow. Annual incidence is 3-4 per 100,000. Infiltration of the marrow by malignant clonal plasma cells commonly results in a normochromic normocytic anaemia (in 70% of patients), but can also cause pancytopenia. The presence of >10% clonal plasma cells in the marrow aspirate, supports the diagnosis. Osteoclast-mediated bone destruction manifesting as bony lytic lesions commonly occur in multiple myeloma and are induced by certain mediators such as the RANK ligand. These result in bone pain, typically back pain, in 60% of patients and hypercalcaemia in 15% of patients.

Serum electrophoresis and urine Bence-Jones protein form key components of the myeloma screen and are positive as a result of the production of monoclonal antibodies from the malignant clonal plasma cells. Excessive monoclonal antibody production can, in < 7% of cases, cause a hyperviscosity syndrome (leading to neurological complaints such as headache, visual disturbances, vertigo and even seizures and coma). Monoclonal paraproteinaemia can also lead to systemic amyloidosis (of the AL type; primary amyloidosis) and acute kidney injury, the latter of which can be exacerbated by hypercalcaemia.

Multiple myeloma must always be excluded in elderly patients presenting with thoracic back pain and a significantly raised ESR. MGUS is the asymptomatic presentation of a triad of paraproteinaemia (< 3g/dL), <10% plasma cells in the bone marrow and absence of end-organ-related damage (bony lytic lesions, hypercalcaemia, anaemia, hyperviscosity and renal insufficiency). It is a premalignant condition with a risk of progression to myeloma at a rate of 1%/year.

Hsu DC, Wilkenfeld P and Joshua DE. Multiple myeloma. British Medical Journal. 2012;344: d7953

17) D. Stop warfarin and give intravenous vitamin K and dried prothrombin complex concentrate

The management of bleeding and raised INR in patients on warfarin is outlined below:

Major bleeding (defined as limb or life-threatening bleeding)

Regardless of INR, all patients with major bleeding should be given dried pro-thrombin complex concentrate (PCC; Beriplex or Octaplex), which completely reverses warfarin-induced anticoagulation in 10 minutes. Beriplex/Octaplex, which are licensed in the UK, consist of concentrated factors II, VII, IX and X. As they have a limited half-life, the shortest being 3-6 hours for factor VII, they should be given in conjunction with 5mg intravenous vitamin K. Fresh Frozen Plasma (FFP) is only used if PCC is not available, as it produces suboptimal reversal of anticoagulation.

Minor bleeding

INR 5.0-8.0 = Stop warfarin, then give IV vitamin K (1-3mg)

INR >8 = Stop warfarin, then give IV vitamin K (1-3mg). If INR is still high after 24 hours, repeat IV vitamin K; 5mg IV vitamin K completely reverses warfarin-induced   anticoagulation.

No Bleeding

INR 5.0-8.0 = Omit one or two doses of warfarin, rechecking INR daily, then give a reduced maintenance dose

INR >8 = Stop warfarin then give oral vitamin K (1-5mg). Repeat vitamin K if INR is still too   high after 24 hours.

British Medical Association and the Royal Pharmaceutical Society of Great Britain. British National Formulary. 62nd ed. UK: BMJ Publishing Group. 2011.

Keeling D, Baglin T, Tait C et al. Guidelines on oral anticoagulation with warfarin – fourth edition. British Journal of Haematology. 2011;154: 311-324

18) B: II, VII, IX, X

By inhibiting the enzyme vitamin K epoxide reductase, warfarin inhibits the carboxylation of gamma glutamic acid residues in clotting factors II, VII, IX and X. These clotting factors normally catalyse the relevant parts of the clotting factor pathways by gliding along the platelet surfaces only after being stabilized by positively charged calcium ions, which essentially act as a bridge between platelets and the clotting factors. The reduced negative charges of the clotting factors, due to their lack of carboxylation, however, prevents their interaction with platelets and thus impairs their function.

Keeling D, Baglin T, Tait C et al. Guidelines on oral anticoagulation with warfarin – fourth edition. British Journal of Haematology. 2011;154: 311-324

19) A: Prolonged aPTT, normal PT, normal TT

The aPTT is a reflection of intrinsic pathway activity, whilst the PT is a reflection of extrinsic pathway activity.

Deficiencies in factor VIII or IX result in isolated prolongation of aPTT. This can be secondary to Haemophilia A (factor VIII deficiency) or B (factor IX deficiency). Von Willebrand factor (vWF) is a carrier of factor VIII, so deficiencies of vWF induce deficiencies of factor VIII, meaning that von Willebrand disease is also associated with an isolated prolongation of the aPTT.

Option B is associated with disseminated intravascular coagulation (DIC), severe hypofibrinogenaemia and advanced liver disease. Option C is associated with heparin contamination.

Isolated prolongation of the prothrombin time (PT) is often due to warfarin therapy. The INR, which is used to monitor the level of anticoagulation, is represented by:

$$INR = (PTtest/PTnormal)^{ISI}$$

The PTtest is the prothrombin time of the test sample, whilst the PTnormal is the prothrombin time of the normal population. ISI is the International Sensitivity Index, and is a number that standardizes the PT measurements by taking into account the variations in the different types of tissue factor produced from different manufacturers.

Triplett DA. Coagulation and Bleeding Disorders: Review and Update. Clinical Chemistry. 2000;46: 1260-9

20) E: Chronic Lymphocytic Leukaemia

Options A to D are recognized causes of massive splenomegaly, whilst option E is associated with moderate splenomegaly. Mild to moderate splenomegaly can also be caused by haemolytic anaemia, infectious mononucleosis and subacute bacterial endocarditis to name a few.

21) A: Imatinib

This patient has chronic myeloid leukaemia (CML), a malignant clonal proliferation of pluripotent stem cells of the myeloid lineage without loss of capacity to differentiate. As with virtually all malignancies, patients commonly present with anaemia and constitutional symptoms such as fatigue, malaise and weight loss. Abdominal discomfort can arise because of splenomegaly, which is potentially massive, extending to at least 5cm below the left costal margin in more than 50% of patients. Bloods often reveal a marked leukocytosis, with basophilia and eosinophilia. Both thrombocytosis and thrombocytopenia can occur.

One of the defining cytogenetic characteristics of CML is the occurrence of a reciprocal translocation between chromosomes 9 and 22 (t(9;22)), which affects nearly 95% of patients. This chromosomal translocation relocates the ABL (Ableson) proto-oncogene (originally on chromosome 9 and encodes a tyrosine kinase enzyme) to the BCR (Breakpoint Cluster Region) on chromosome 22. The resulting Philadelphia chromosome (transformed chromosome 22) carries the BCR-ABL gene, which encodes a constitutively active tyrosine kinase, ultimately giving rise to the CML phenotype. Imatinib was among the first selective tyrosine kinase inhibitors targeting this BCR-ABL fusion protein, and has revolutionized the treatment of this condition.

Quintas-Cardama A and Cortes JE. Chronic Myeloid Leukemia: Diagnosis and Treatment. Mayo Clinic Proceedings. 2006;81: 973-88.

22) A: ATRA and arsenic trioxide

Acute myeloid leukaemia M3 is also known as acute promyelocytic leukaemia (APL). It is characterized by a t(15;17) chromosomal translocation that results in the formation of the fusion protein PML-RARalpha, which inhibits differentiation, and promotes the proliferation of immature leukaemic myeloid cells. The development of All-Trans Retinoic Acid (ATRA) has completely revolutionized the treatment of APL and functions by inducing the differentiation of the abnormal myeloid precursor cells and triggers transient remissions. Arsenic trioxide works synergistically by promoting apoptosis of the leukaemic cells.

de Thé H and Chen Z. Acute promyelocytic leukaemia: novel insights into the mechanisms of cure. Nature Reviews: Cancer. 2010;7: 775-83

23) B: t(8;14)

The following outlines some key chromosomal translocations and their associated conditions:

a) t(9;22) and chronic myeloid leukaemia (BCR-ABL fusion)
b) t(8;14) and Burkitt's lymphoma (cMYC mutation)
c) t(15;17) and acute promyelocytic leukaemia (PML-RARalpha fusion)
d) t(14;18) and follicular lymphoma
e) t(11;14) and mantle cell lymphoma (overexpression of cyclin D1)

24) C: JAK-2

Polycythaemia rubra vera (PRV), also known as primary polycythaemia, is a clonal myeloproliferative disorder characterized by excessive production of erythrocytes from the bone marrow, leading to increased total red blood cell volume, and an inordinately high haematocrit and haemoglobin. Patients often suffer from hyperviscosity symptoms such as headache, tinnitus, vertigo, visual disturbances, angina and intermittent claudication. Patients are at increased risk from arterial and venous thrombotic (strokes, TIA, MI, DVT and PE) and haemorrhagic complications (usually epistaxis and gum bleeding, but also GI bleeding). Patients often have high histamine levels, rendering them at increased risk of peptic ulcer disease and pruritus particularly worse after hot baths and showers. Erythromelalgia describes the intense episodic burning sensations, erythema and swelling of the hands or feet. PRV is often due to JAK-2 mutations.

Secondary polycythaemia is increased haematocrit, usually secondary to chronic hypoxaemia (e.g. in heavy smokers with COPD) or secondary to increased erythropoietin secretion from renal or hepatic cysts or renal cell carcinoma for example. Apparent polycythaemia is a relative increase in haematocrit due to a contracted plasma volume. Gaisbock's syndrome is apparent polycythaemia that typically occurs in sedentary overweight male patients with hypertension.

Tefferi A. Polycythemia Vera: A Comprehensive Review and Clinical Recommendations. Mayo Clinic Proceedings. 2003; 78:174-94

25) E: Stage IIIb

The presence of Reed Sternberg cells is characteristic of Hodgkin's lymphoma. Patients commonly present with lymphadenopathy, which may be accompanied by 'B' symptoms. B symptoms include fever, night sweats and weight loss (more than 10% within the previous 6 months).

Patients with Hodgkin's lymphoma can be staged using the Ann Arbor classification, which is as follows:

Stage I = lymphadenopathy of one lymph node area
Stage II = lymphadenopathy of two or more lymph node areas on the same side of the diaphragm
Stage III = lymphadenopathy of two or more lymph node areas on opposite sides of the diaphragm
Stage IV = Disseminated disease with involvement of the liver and/or bone marrow

In the presence of B symptoms, the suffix b should be added to the stage number.

26) E: Iron deficiency

This patient has a macrocytic anaemia, which can be caused by alcoholism and options A to D. Iron deficiency causes a microcytic anaemia.

B12 and folate deficiency specifically cause a megaloblastic anaemia due to interrupted DNA synthesis. A bone marrow aspirate typically reveals abnormally large precursor cells called megaloblasts. B12 and folate deficiency can also potentially cause a pancytopenia and the presence of hypersegmented neutrophils. Vitamin B12 is absorbed in the terminal ileum once bound to intrinsic factor, which is produced by the gastric parietal cells. Therefore, any condition that disrupts the production of intrinsic factor (e.g. pernicious anaemia where there is autoimmune destruction of the intrinsic factor producing cells) or pathologically affects the terminal ileum (e.g. inflammatory bowel disease) can impair vitamin B12 absorption.

B12 deficiency can also be associated with neurological compromise, such as peripheral neuropathy, or in severe cases, subacute combined degeneration of the cord; the latter can manifest as ataxia and loss of proprioceptive function due to loss of the integrity of lateral and dorsal white matter columns, respectively.

Haemolytic anaemia can be associated with normocytosis or macrocytosis, depending on the amount of reticulocyte production (as reticulocytes have 1.5 times the MCV of red cells).

Aslinia F, Mazza JJ and Yale SH. Megaloblastic Anemia and Other Causes of Macrocytosis. Clinical Medicine & Research. 2006; 4:236-41

Dermatology Questions

1) Which of the following is the most common identifiable cause of erythema nodosum?

A. Tuberculosis
B. Sarcoidosis
C. Sulfonamides
D. Streptococcal infection
E. Ulcerative colitis

2) A 28-year old male presents to his GP as over the past 3 months he has developed a rash on both his elbows and knees.

On examination, there are large, well-delineated erythematous plaques with overlying silvery scale.

What is the most likely diagnosis?

A. Psoriasis
B. Eczema
C. Contact dermatitis
D. Erythema multiforme
E. Mycosis fungoides

3) A 34-year old female with chronic plaque psoriasis is reviewed in the dermatology clinic. She has failed to respond to multiple different topical preparations including courses of potent topical steroids and vitamin D analogues.

What is the next most appropriate management?

A. Methotrexate
B. Ciclosporin
C. PUVA
D. Narrow band UV-B
E. Acitretin

4) A 62-year old lady presents to her GP as she has noticed a progressive change in colour of her right axilla.

On examination, there is a large hyperpigmented plaque with a velvety appearance.

Which of the following malignancies is this dermatosis most strongly associated with?

A. Small cell lung carcinoma
B. Non small cell lung carcinoma
C. Anaplastic thyroid carcinoma
D. Gastric adenocarcinoma
E. Colon adenocarcinoma

5) A 24-year old male student presents with a 4 day history of rash.

On examination, there are numerous macules, papules and target lesions principally affecting the extremities.

Which of the following is the most likely aetiological agent?

A. Herpes simplex virus
B. Epstein-Barr virus
C. Mycoplasma pneumoniae
D. Sulfonamide
E. Penicillin

6) A 28-year old lady with epilepsy presents to the emergency department with a 3-day history of rash, fever and painful erosions affecting her eyes, mouth and vagina.

On examination, the patient looks generally unwell with a generalised maculopapular rash, target lesions and bullae, collectively affecting nearly 10% of her body surface area.

What is the most likely diagnosis?

A. Erythema multiforme
B. Toxic epidermal necrolysis
C. Stevens-Johnson syndrome
D. Erythroderma
E. Erythema toxicum

7) A 64-year old male presents with a 4-month history of a pruritic, migratory rash in association with haemoptysis and weight loss.

On examination, there are multiple erythematous skin lesions on his upper trunk and shoulders that follow a pattern of concentric, serpiginous raised bands.

What is the most likely diagnosis?

A. Erythema chronicum migrans
B. Erythema gyratum repens
C. Erythema ab igne
D. Erythema multiforme
E. Erythema marginatum

8) Which of the following statements regarding atopic dermatitis is FALSE?

A. It is often associated with asthma and allergic rhinitis
B. Concordance rate of dizygotic twins is 15%
C. Spongiosis and a perivascular lymphoid infiltrate is the histologic hallmark of acute eczematous lesions
D. It typically affects the flexural surfaces of the limbs
E. 5-10% of children are affected

9) Which of the following is the most potent topical corticosteroid?

A. Hydrocortisone
B. Dermovate
C. Eumovate
D. Epaderm
E. Betnovate

10) A 54-year old male patient presents to his GP with a very painful lesion on his right leg that has progressed rapidly over the past 2 days. This has occurred in association with malaise, generalised arthralgia and myalgia.

On examination, there is a large deep ulcer, with mucopurulent exudate, undermining a well-defined violaceous border. The surrounding skin is erythematous and indurated.

Which of the following is this skin condition most strongly associated with?

A. Multiple myeloma
B. Rheumatoid arthritis
C. Acute myeloid leukaemia
D. Behcet's disease
E. Inflammatory bowel disease

11) Scraping psoriatic plaques reveals punctate haemorrhages.

What is the name given to this sign?

A. Koebnerization
B. Hutchinson's sign
C. Nikolsky's sign
D. Russell's sign
E. Auspitz sign

12) A 28-year old female with coeliac disease presents with a highly pruritic vesicular skin eruption affecting both her elbows.

What is the first line drug treatment?

A. Dapsone
B. Ciclosporin
C. Prednisolone
D. Azathioprine
E. Colchicine

13) A 75-year old gentleman presents to the emergency department with a generalised eruption of skin blisters.

On examination, there are numerous tense, fluid-filled blisters on the lower abdomen, flexural surfaces of the arms and the anterior thighs. Nikolsky sign is negative.

Immunoblotting is negative for anti-type VII collagen antibodies.

What is the most likely diagnosis?

A. Pemphigus vulgaris
B. Pemphigus foliaceus
C. Bullous pemphigoid
D. Dermatitis herpetiformis
E. Epidermolysis bullosa acquisita

14) A 22-year old male rugby player presents to his GP with a highly pruritic rash on his right arm.

On examination, there is a localised annular lesion measuring 3cm in diameter. The lesion has a raised, erythematous, scaling edge with a central clearing.

What is the most appropriate investigation?

A. Woods lamp
B. Excisional biopsy
C. Incisional biopsy
D. Dermatoscopy
E. Skin scrapings for microscopy and culture

15) A 48-year old male with longstanding type II diabetes presents with a papular eruption on the dorsum of his left hand.

On examination, there is a small localised group of erythematous papules arranged in a circle, around a central, clear depressed area.

What is the most likely diagnosis?

A. Granuloma annulare
A. Tinea corpora
B. Tinea manuum
C. Necrobiosis lipoidica diabeticorum
D. Staphylococcal skin infection

16) Which of the following statements regarding malignant melanoma is FALSE?

A. Radial size is the most important prognostic parameter
B. Superficial spreading melanoma is the most common subtype
C. Melanoma accounts for approximately 4% of all skin cancers
D. CDKNA2 mutations is the most common cause of inherited melanomas
E. Melanomas more frequently metastasise to the lungs than the brain

17) A 35-year old Caucasian female presents to her GP with a rash on her arms.

On examination, there are multiple pink, dome-shaped lesions ranging from 2-5mm in diameter with umbilicated centres.

What is the most likely underlying cause for this presentation?

A. Herpes Simplex virus
B. Cytomegalovirus
C. Streptococci
D. Pox virus
E. HIV

18) A 46-year old male with a history of hepatitis C presents to his GP with an intensely pruritic rash on both wrists.

On examination, there are numerous violaceous, polygonal, papular lesions on the volar surfaces of both wrists.

What is the most likely diagnosis?

A. Lichen planus
B. Lichen sclerosus
C. Pityriasis rosea
D. Pityriasis versicolor
E. Atopic dermatitis

19) A 68-year old male farmer presents with a small lesion on the side of his nose.

On examination, there is a small nodule with a rolled border, pearly appearance and overlying telangiectasia.

What is the most likely diagnosis?

A. Squamous cell carcinoma
B. Amelanotic melanoma
C. Bowen's disease
D. Keratoacanthoma
E. Basal cell carcinoma

20) An 18-year old female on isotretinoin for severe acne is reviewed in the dermatology clinic.

Which of the following does not need to be monitored during the course of treatment?

A. Liver function tests
B. Serum lipids
C. Contraceptive status
D. Full blood count
E. Blood pressure

Dermatology Answers

1)   D: Streptococcal infection

Erythema nodosum often presents as painful, tender, red subcutaneous nodules, symmetrically located on the anterior surface of the shins, although they can also occur on the extensor surfaces of the elbows, thighs and trunk. It is a form of panniculitis whereby there is septal inflammation of the subcutaneous fat, thought to be due to a type IV hypersensitivity reaction to various antigens. The lesions are poorly demarcated, do not ulcerate, and after fading into a bruise-like appearance, tend to heal completely by 1 to 2 months.

Although erythema nodosum is most commonly idiopathic, it is frequently a manifestation of systemic disease. When an underlying cause is identified, it is most likely to be secondary to streptococcal throat infection, though many other possible causes are recognised. These include inflammatory bowel disease (ulcerative colitis being more strongly associated with erythema nodosum than Crohn's disease), tuberculosis, sarcoidosis, drugs (e.g. sulphonamides and the oral contraceptive pill), malignancy (typically lymphoma or leukaemia) and Behcet's disease.

Treatment involves managing the underlying condition, bed rest and unless contraindicated, NSAIDs.

Schwartz RA and Nervi SJ. Erythema Nodosum: A Sign of Systemic Disease. American Family Physician. 2007; 75: 695-700.

2)   A: Psoriasis

Psoriasis is a chronic inflammatory, relapsing and remitting skin disease. It has a prevalence of 1.3-2.2% in the UK and is a major cause of psychological and social morbidity. Chronic plaque psoriasis, with which this patient presents, is the most common variant and accounts for around 90% of cases of psoriasis. Plaques may be itchy and most commonly affect the extensor surfaces of the limbs (usually the knees and elbows), the scalp and the lower back; in some cases, the flexural surfaces can be involved.

Other subtypes include:

a) *Guttate psoriasis* - typically follows an upper respiratory tract infection in young adults. It presents as an eruption of salmon-pink papules on the upper trunk and proximal limbs.
b) *Generalised pustular psoriasis* – often preceded by constitutional symptoms including headache, fever, chills and arthralgia. This is followed by a generalised eruption of pustules principally affecting the flexural surfaces and the anogenital areas. The pustules coalesce, dry out and then desquamate in sheets leaving behind a raw erythematous skin surface.
c) *Erythrodermic psoriasis* – erythroderma can occur secondary to any exfoliative dermatitis and can be caused by psoriasis, eczema or drug-induced skin reactions. It is a dermatological emergency and occurs when more than 90% of the skin surface is affected by an exfoliative dermatitis. Patients are at risk of hypothermia, dehydration, sepsis and high output cardiac failure.

Smith CH and Barker JNWN. Psoriasis and its management. British Medical Journal. 2006; 333:380-4.

3) D: Narrow band UV-B

Chronic plaque psoriasis should initially be managed with topical treatments. This may include short-term intermittent courses of potent to very potent topical steroids. Long-term use is not recommended due to the side effects of skin atrophy, striae and the increased likelihood for rebound of the psoriasis (or whichever underlying skin condition is being treated) shortly after stopping the long-term steroid treatment. Topical vitamin D analogues such as calcipotriol, calcitriol and tacalcitol, however, are recommended for long-term treatment due to the absence of such side effects. Other topical treatments include short-contact dithranol treatment, coal tar preparations, salicylic acid and coconut oils, the latter three being commonly employed in scalp psoriasis.

Failure to respond to topical therapies requires stepping up treatment to narrow band UV-B phototherapy. PUVA is an alternative but not recommended as next-line treatment if topical therapy fails.

PUVA involves topical or oral administration of Psoralens (a photosensitising agent) followed by Ultraviolet-A exposure.

Severe psoriasis refractory to the aforementioned treatments will require systemic therapy with methotrexate, ciclosporin or acitretin, and if these fail, biological treatment (e.g. anti-TNF monoclonal antibodies).

Scottish Intercollegiate Guidelines Network. Diagnosis and management of psoriasis and psoriatic arthritis in adults. SIGN guideline 121.

4) D: Gastric adenocarcinoma

This patient has acanthosis nigricans, which is most commonly found on the axilla, posterior neck or groin. Although frequently associated with obesity and insulin-resistance, it can be a dermatological paraneoplastic phenomenon of underlying malignancy, of which gastric adenocarcinomas are the most likely culprit.

Higgins SP, Freemark M, Prose NS. Acanthosis nigricans: a practical approach to evaluation and management. Dermatology Online Journal. 2008;14: 2.

5) A: Herpes simplex virus

The most likely diagnosis is erythema multiforme. It is an acute self-limiting skin condition thought to arise secondary to a hypersensitivity reaction in response to certain drugs or infections. The most common identifiable cause is Herpes Simplex virus infection, which accounts for more than 50% of cases. Other causes include Mycoplasma pneumonia and fungal infections as well as penicillins, NSAIDs and sulphonamides. The rash typically affects young adults aged 20 to 40. During its natural course, it begins symmetrically in the extremities as multiple sharply demarcated pink macules and papules, which then spread proximally.

The papules subsequently enlarge and their central portions become darker red and purpuric. Characteristic target lesions thus develop, which have a regular round shape, a central darker red area, a paler pink or oedematous zone and an outermost red ring. The rash then resolves spontaneously over a period of 3 to 5 weeks.

Lamoreux MR and Sternbach MR. Erythema Multiforme. American Family Physician. 2006;74: 1883-8.

6) **C: Stevens-Johnson syndrome**

Stevens-Johnson syndrome (SJS) is a severe form of erythema multiforme with involvement of the mucous membranes. It commonly occurs secondary to various infections (including group A-haemolytic streptococci, mycoplasma and influenza) and drugs (most commonly antibiotics, typically penicillins and sulfa drugs, and anticonvulsants). This patient has probably developed SJS as a result of exposure to anticonvulsants given her history of epilepsy. Toxic-epidermal necrolysis (TEN) is a more severe variant of SJS in which there is at least 30% epidermal detachment (SJS is defined by <10%). Patients with TEN are profoundly unwell, presenting with large patches of desquamation, clinically mimicking severe burns.

Gerull R, Nelle M and Schaible T. Toxic epidermal necrolysis and Stevens-Johnson syndrome: A review. Critical Care Medicine. 2011;39: 1-12

Fein JD and Hamann KL. Stevens-Johnson Syndrome. The New England Journal of Medicine. 2005;352: 1696.

7) **B: Erythema gyratum repens**

Erythema gyratum repens is a highly characteristic, rare rash that, in up to 80% of cases, is a dermatological manifestation of underlying malignancy. It is most strongly associated with lung cancer, followed by oesophageal and breast cancers.

Erythema chronicum migrans is the classical 'bullseye' rash associated with Lyme disease. Erythema ab igne is the reticular rash induced by long-term exposure to heat (e.g. hot water bottle). Erythema multiforme is described in question 5. Erythema marginatum is the rash associated with acute rheumatic fever and represents one of the major Jones criteria.

Delage M and Naouri M. Erythema Gyratum Repens. The New England Journal of Medicine. 2010;362: 1814

8) **E: 5-10% of children are affected**

Eczema (also known as atopic dermatitis) is a common, chronic, relapsing-remitting, dry, itchy, inflammatory skin condition affecting 2-10% of adults and 15-30% of children. Both genetic and environmental factors are implicated in the pathogenesis of the disease. This is supported by twin studies, which have shown that the concordance rate amongst dizygotic twins is 15% and in monozygotic twins 77%.

During infancy, eczema has a predilection for affecting the cheeks and scalp. Later during childhood and adulthood, the lesions typically affect the flexural surfaces, although in many cases, children grow out of eczema. The eczematous lesions are very itchy, and after a chronic period of rubbing and itching, they eventually form thickened, lichenified plaques. Eczema is often associated with other atopic conditions, which include asthma and allergic rhinitis.

Management requires avoidance of soaps, detergents and perfumes, which can trigger flare-ups of eczema, and regular liberal use of emollients (e.g. diprobase, 50/50 cream, epaderm). During flare-ups, on top of these usual treatments, patients should be offered short-term courses of topical steroids. In severe cases refractory to potent/very potent topical steroids, second-line treatments include the topical immunomodulators tacrolimus and pimecrolimus (calcineurin inhibitors). Alternative treatments for severe eczema in adults include phototherapy (PUVA or narrow band UV-B) or systemic treatment with methotrexate, ciclosporin or azathioprine.

Bieber T. Atopic Dermatitis. The New England Journal of Medicine. 2008;358: 1483-94

9) B: Dermovate

Epaderm is an emollient, not a topical steroid. The potency of the remaining steroid preparations (brand names) can be remembered by recalling the phrase 'Help Every Budding Dermatologist' for Hydrocortisone, Eumovate, Betnovate and Dermovate. These correspond, respectively, to mild, moderate, potent and very potent topical steroids.

When applying topical steroids, it is useful to work in terms of fingertip units. Each fingertip unit (corresponding to a strand of cream or ointment extending from the tip of the finger to the proximal nail fold) should be used to cover a surface area equivalent to two handprints. This helps to prevent excessive use of topical steroids, thereby reducing the incidence of side effects (e.g. skin atrophy and striae).

Brown S and Reynolds NJ. Atopic and non-atopic eczema. British Medical Journal. 2006; 332: 584-8.

10) E: Inflammatory bowel disease

The description is typical of classic pyoderma gangrenosum, a rare non-infectious neutrophilic dermatosis. It most commonly affects the shins and often begins as a group of sterile pustules that rapidly progress over 24-48 hours, ulcerating and coalescing into a single deep, very painful, ulcer with undermined violaceous borders. It is associated with systemic disease in nearly 50% of cases, most commonly inflammatory bowel disease (both Crohn's and ulcerative colitis). All the remaining answer options are examples of other less commonly associated systemic conditions.

Treatment is notoriously difficult, requiring good local wound care supplemented with high dose systemic steroids and/or immunosuppressants.

Wollina U. Pyoderma gangrenosum – a review. Orphanet journal of Rare Diseases. 2007; 2: 19

Brooklyn T, Dunnill G and Probert C. Diagnosis and treatment of pyoderma gangrenosum. British Medical Journal. 2006;333: 181-4

11) E: Auspitz sign

The correct answer is Auspitz sign. Koebnerization (or Koebner phenomenon) refers to the formation of new skin lesions along lines of trauma and can occur in psoriasis, vitiligo or lichen planus amongst other conditions.

Nikolsky's sign is elicited by applying tangential pressure to the skin. The formation of a blister is positive for this sign and occurs in pemphigus (but not bullous pemphigoid), toxic epidermal necrolysis and staphylococcal scalded skin syndrome.

Russell's sign refers to the callosities of the knuckles resulting from repeated episodes of self-induced vomiting, typically occurring in bulimia.

Hutchinson's sign can either refer to the melanonychia in subungual melanoma or the formation of papulo-vesicular lesions on the tip of the nose in herpes zoster ophthalmicus, heralding impending ipsilateral corneal involvement.

Madke, B and Nayak C. Eponymous signs in dermatology. Indian Dermatology Online Journal. 2012;3: 159-65.

12) A: Dapsone

This patient has dermatitis herpetiformis, a highly pruritic autoimmune skin eruption strongly associated with gluten-sensitive enteropathy. It preferentially affects the extensor surfaces (knees, hips and buttocks). Immunohistochemical stains characteristically show IgA and C3 deposits clustered in the dermal papillae.

After adhering to a gluten-free diet, first line treatment is with dapsone. In patients at risk of haemolysis, such as those with G6PD deficiency, dapsone should be avoided and replaced with sulfapyridine instead. Less effective alternative treatments encompass immunosuppressants and steroids, including those listed amongst the answer options.

Sticherling M and Erfurt-Berge C. Autoimmune blistering diseases of the skin. Autoimmunity Reviews. 2012;11: 226-30.

13) C: Bullous pemphigoid

Bullous pemphigoid, pemphigus and epidermolysis bullosa (EB) acquisita are all auto-immune blistering conditions of the skin. Bullous pemphigoid is characterised by the production of auto-antibodies targeting the hemidesmosomal structures, which normally anchor the basal epidermal keratinocytes to the underlying basement membrane. This results in the separation of cells at the dermal-epidermal junction leading to the formation of tense, subepidermal fluid-filled blisters.

Pemphigus, however, is characterised by the production of anti-desmosomal antibodies, which anchor the network of epidermal keratinocytes together. Destruction of the desmosomes leads to acantholysis and the formation of flaccid, intra-epidermal, fluid-filled blisters. Several variants exist, of which pemphigus vulgaris is the most severe and most common.

The clinical presentations of EB acquisita and bullous pemphigoid are very similar, both being sub-epidermal blistering diseases. The two can be distinguished on the basis of positivity for anti-type VII collagen antibodies in EB acquisita, which drives the pathogenesis of the disease. The two can further be distinguished via indirect immunofluorescence studies on salt-split skin. Circulating IgG antibodies of EB acquisita sera bind to the dermal side of the split, whereas antibodies from bullous pemphigoid sera bind to the epidermal side.

Cotell S, Robinson ND and Lawrence SC. Autoimmune Blistering Skin Diseases. The American Journal of Emergency Medicine. 2000; 18: 288-99.

14) E: Skin scrapings for microscopy and culture

Fungi that cause skin infections are collectively grouped as dermatophytes and include Trichophyton, Microsporum and Epidermophyton species. The description in the question stem is the typical clinical finding in someone with dermatophytosis.

It is spread through direct skin contact or via fomites and has an incubation period of about 1-3 weeks. Once infection has started, it grows in a centrifugal pattern, creating an evolving scaly annular plaque with a central clearing; this ring-like appearance has earned it the name 'ringworm' albeit a misnomer as they're not caused by worms. Dermatophytosis can be grouped according to the location of the body affected, as follows:

1) Tinea capitis – scalp
2) Tinea corporis – trunk
3) Tinea cruris –groin
4) Tinea manuum – hand
5) Tinea pedis – foot (i.e. athletes foot)

To make a diagnosis, skin scrapings for microscopy and culture should be taken. Wood's lamp is not a specific test for fungal skin infection.

Treatment usually includes topical anti-fungals such as topical allylamines (e.g. terbinafine) or the topical azoles (e.g. ketoconazole, clotrimazole or miconazole).

Fungal nail infections (onychomycosis) fail to resolve with topical therapy, as they are unable to sufficiently penetrate the nail plate. Thus, they often require treatment with oral antifungals such as oral terbinafine or itraconazole.

Weinstein A and Berman B. Topical Treatment of Common Superficial Tinea infections. American Family Physician. 2002; 15: 2095-103.

15) A: Granuloma annulare

Patients with diabetes are at risk of all the conditions in the answer options. The description however is most consistent with granuloma annulare. Necrobiosis lipoidica diabeticorum is a rare, necrotising, granulomatous skin disease affecting around 0.3% of diabetics. It initially develops as an erythematous plaque, typically on the shins, the centre of which then gradually turns into a yellow waxy appearance.

Perez I and Kohn R. Cutaneous manifestations of diabetes. Journal of the American Academy of Dermatology. 1994;30:519-31

16) A: Radial size is the most important prognostic parameter

Despite accounting for only 4% of all dermatological malignancies, malignant melanoma is responsible for 80% of all deaths from skin cancer. They are the most aggressive forms of skin cancer and require early detection and treatment in order to minimise mortality. Several different subtypes exist including:

1) Superficial spreading melanoma – most common subtype accounting for 70% of all cutaneous malignant melanomas
2) Nodular melanoma – accounts for 10-15% of melanomas and one of the most aggressive subtype
3) Acral lentiginous melanomas – occurs on glabrous skin including the palms, soles and subungual areas. In the latter case, they can be mistaken for bruises.
4) Lentigo maligna melanoma – these arise when melanoma in situ (also known as Hutchinson's melanotic freckle) becomes invasive.
5) Mucosal lentiginous melanoma – a rare form of melanoma that arises in mucosal epithelia (e.g. respiratory, gastrointestinal and genitourinary tracts).

In order to detect melanomas, it is useful to use the ABCDE rule, which outlines features of the skin lesion that make the probability of melanoma high.

A – Asymmetry: is the lesion asymmetrical?
B – Border: does it have irregular borders?
C – Colour: is the pigmentation dark and heterogenous (i.e. multiple shades   of tan, brown or black)?
D- Diameter: is it more than 6 mm?
E – Evolution: has the lesion changed in colour, size or shape rapidly over time?

Skin lesions that are asymmetrical, have irregular borders, heterogenous and dark in pigmentation, a diameter of more than 6mm and have changed quite quickly over time are most likely to represent malignant melanomas.

The thickness, not the diameter, of the lesion is the most important prognostic predictor and is central to Breslow's and Clark's classification.

Shenenberger DW. Cutaneous Malignant Melanoma: A Primary Care Perspective. American Family Physician. 2012;85: 161-8.

Miller AJ and Mihm Jr MC. Melanoma. The New England Journal of Medicine. 2006; 355: 51-65

17) D: Pox virus

The presentation is typical of Molluscum contagiosum, a self-limiting, relatively harmless skin infection caused by the Pox virus.

18) A: Lichen planus

The diagnosis is Lichen planus. Although the aetiology is unclear, there is a recognised association with hepatitis C virus infection. The rash typically affects the distal extremities but can also involve the genitalia and mucous membranes.

Lichen sclerosus typically affects the genital and anal areas, beginning as shiny, white polygonal papules that coalesce into plaques. The rash frequently itches, but can also cause pain and discomfort. The aetiology is unclear.

Pityriasis rosea is an erythematous rash, often preceded by an upper respiratory tract infection, which begins as an isolated pink oval or round 'herald patch' classically on the abdomen. One to two weeks later, the rash becomes symmetrically generalised on the torso and abdomen, adopting a 'christmas tree' distribution, following the lines of skin cleavage (Langers lines).

Pityriasis versicolor is a rash caused by the overgrowth of Pityrosporum orbiculare (Malassezia furfur), a fungus that forms part of the normal skin flora. It is a benign condition characterised by multiple well-demarcated macules and patches most frequently on the trunk, back and abdomen. The rash is hyperpigmented in patients with lighter skin colours and hypopigmented in those with darker skin colours.

Shengyuan L, Songpo Y, Wen W, Wenjing T, Haitao Z and Binyou W. Hepatitis C virus and lichen planus: a reciprocal association determined by a meta-analysis. Archives of Dermatology. 2009;145:1040-7.

19) E: Basal cell carcinoma

As with all skin cancers, basal cell carcinomas (BCC) most commonly occur on sun-exposed areas of the body. Although BCCs very rarely metastasise, they should be excised early, as they will otherwise continue to grow and invade surrounding structures (hence their nickname 'rodent ulcers'). Multiple variants of BCC are recognised:

1) *Nodular BCC* – this is described in the question stem and represents the most common variant.
2) *Superficial BCC* – this presents as a scaly erythematous patch or plaque and can be difficult to distinguish clinically from a squamous cell carcinoma (SCC)
3) *Morpheaform BCC* – this presents as a whitish scar-like appearance with poorly demarcated margins and can go unrecognised for years.

Squamous cell carcinomas can take on variable appearances, but frequently include erythematous papules or plaques that ulcerate and bleed. They are more likely to metastasise than BCCs, but are not as aggressive as melanomas. Multiple precursors have been identified and include:

1) Actinic keratosis – these are indurated scaly lesions typically 2-6mm in diameter and unless treated early (e.g. with cryosurgery or topical fluorouracil), can develop invasive potential.

2) Bowen's disease – this most commonly develops on the shins and represents squamous cell carcinoma in-situ (higher grade than actinic keratosis). Appearances can be difficult to distinguish from invasive squamous cell carcinoma and superficial BCC.

3) Erythroplasia of Queyrat – another form of squamous carcinoma in-situ, it occurs on the glans penis and is less common than Bowen's disease.

Keratoacanthomas are well known to mimic SCCs. They are relatively common low-grade tumours originating from the pilosebaceous units. They can be distinguished from SCCs by their more rapid growth pattern (few weeks), their spontaneous resolution (over a few months), and their characteristic central keratin plugs, which classically project like horns.

Treatment of BCCs and SCCs usually requires surgical excision. If maximum tissue conservation is essential, then modern techniques such as Moh's micrographic surgery can be employed to allow precise control of excision margins.

Rubin AI, Chen EH and Ratner D. Basal-Cell Carcinoma. The New England Journal of Medicine. 2005;353: 2262-9.

Alam M and Ratner D. Cutaneous Squamous-Cell Carcinoma. The New England Journal of Medicine. 2001; 344: 975-83

20) E: Blood pressure

Isotretinoin is a vitamin A derivative used to treat severe acne. It is highly teratogenic explaining why all women of child-bearing age must have adequate contraception in place. Patients are also at risk of raised serum cholesterol and triglycerides, transaminases and agranulocytosis, explaining why serum lipids, liver function tests and full blood count should, respectively, be monitored. Hypertension is not a well-recognised side effect of isotretinoin.

British Medical Association and the Royal Pharmaceutical Society of Great Britain. British National Formulary. 62nd edition. UK: BMJ Publishing Group. 2011.

Ophthalmology Questions

1) A 64-year old gentleman presents to the emergency eye clinic with a 3-hour history of sudden onset right sided eye pain accompanied by blurring of vision and seeing haloes.

   On examination, there is scleral injection of the right eye, corneal haze, reduced visual acuity to 6/60 and a fixed mid-dilated pupil.

   Which of the following is NOT an appropriate treatment?

   A. IV acetazolamide
   B. Topical steroids
   C. Topical timolol
   D. Topical pilocarpine
   E. Topical Tropicamide

2) Which of the following is NOT a recognised sign of open angle glaucoma?

   A. Cup:disc ratio of 0.8
   B. Peripapillary atrophy
   C. Vessel bayoneting
   D. AV nipping
   E. Notching of the neuroretinal rim

3) A hypertensive patient is examined in the ophthalmology clinic.

   On fundoscopy examination, there is silver wiring, AV nipping, cotton wool spots and flame shaped haemorrhages.

   What grade hypertensive retinopathy does this represent?

   A. Grade 1
   B. Grade 2
   C. Grade 3
   D. Grade 4
   E. Grade 5

4) A 62-year old male presents to the emergency department with sudden onset, painless loss of vision affecting his left eye.

Past medical history includes ischaemic heart disease and previous TIAs.

On examination, visual acuity is reduced to counting fingers for the left eye, but normal 6/6 acuity for the right eye. Fundoscopy of the left eye reveals a pale retina with a cherry red spot.

What is the most likely diagnosis?

A. Central retinal artery occlusion
B. Branch retinal artery occlusion
C. Central retinal vein occlusion
D. Anterior ischaemic optic neuropathy
E. Wet age-related macular degeneration

5) A 50-year old gentleman presents to the emergency eye clinic with sudden onset painless loss of vision of the right eye shortly after waking.

He denies a recent history of headache.

On examination, visual acuity is 6/60 on the right, but 6/5 on the left. There is a relative inferior visual altitudinal defect. Fundoscopy of the left eye reveals a cup-to-disc ratio of 0.2.

What is the most likely diagnosis?

A. Arteritic anterior ischaemic optic neuropathy
B. Non-arteritic anterior ischaemic optic neuropathy
C. Hemi-central vein retinal occlusion
D. Optic neuritis
E. Posterior ischaemic optic neuropathy

6) Which of the following is NOT a recognised cause of a Marcus Gunn pupil?

A. Optic neuritis
B. Anterior ischaemic optic neuropathy
C. Central retinal artery occlusion
D. Optic tumour
E. Vitreous haemorrhage

7) Which of the following treatments have been proven to slow down the rate of wet age-related macular degeneration?

A. Rituximab
B. Etarnecept
C. Adalimumab
D. Ranibizumab
E. Infliximab

8) A 28-year old businessman presents with a 2-day history of right eye pain, photophobia and blurred vision.

Fluorescein dye staining shows a dendritic ulcer.

What is the most likely causative organism?

A. Toxoplasma Gondii
B. Cytomegalovirus (CMV)
C. Herpes simplex virus (HSV)
D. Varicella zoster virus (VZV)
E. Epstein Barr virus (EBV)

9) A 12-year old boy is brought to see the GP by his mother who reports her concerns that her son 'keeps bumping into things.' She also states that he has had a chronic severe difficulty performing most tasks in dimly lit places.

On examination, there is loss of the peripheral visual field. Fundoscopy shows a bony spiculated appearance.

Which of the following is NOT associated with this condition?

A. Usher syndrome
B. Kearns-Sayre syndrome
C. Abetalipoproteinaemia
D. Refsum's disease
E. Marfan's syndrome

10) A 42-year old lady presents to her GP with a 2-day history of a red right eye. She complains of a gritty and itchy sensation and that her right eyelid has tended to stick together, especially in the mornings.

On examination, there is a purulent discharge from the right eye. Visual acuity, fields and pupillary response to light are all normal.

What is the most likely diagnosis?

A. Viral conjunctivitis
B. Bacterial conjunctivitis
C. Allergic conjunctivitis
D. Anterior uveitis
E. Acute angle closure glaucoma

11) A 62-year old gentleman with myopia suddenly noticed flashes of light in his left eye, which started 2 days ago. A day later, he noticed floaters, which was shortly followed by progressive loss of vision that gradually swept across part of his visual field.

Which of the following is the most likely diagnosis?

A. Retinal detachment
B. Posterior vitreous detachment
C. Wet age-related macular degeneration
D. Posterior uveitis
E. Cataracts

12) A 24-year old male presents with an acutely painful red eye and photophobia.

On examination, there is peri-limbal injection and an irregularly shaped pupil poorly reactive to light.

Which of the following conditions is least commonly associated with this acute eye pathology?

A. Ankylosing spondylitis
B. Reactive arthritis
C. Psoriatic arthritis
D. Ulcerative colitis
E. Rheumatoid arthritis

13) Which of the following is NOT a feature of pre-proliferative diabetic retinopathy?

A. Cotton wool spots
B. Intra-retinal microvascular abnormalities (IRMAs)
C. Vitreous haemorrhage
D. Hard exudates
E. Venous beading

14) A 54-year old gentleman presents with a 3-week history of progressive blurring of vision of his right eye.

He is known to suffer from AIDS, which was diagnosed 15 years previously.

His most recent CD4 count 2 months ago was 40 cells/mm^3

Examination of the right fundus reveals the 'pizza pie' sign.

What is the MOST likely diagnosis?

A. Posterior uveitis secondary to Toxoplasmosis
B. Posterior uveitis secondary to Cryptococcus
C. Retinitis secondary to Human Immunodeficiency Virus (HIV)
D. Retinitis secondary to Cytomegalovirus (CMV)
E. Retinitis secondary to Varicella Zoster Virus (VZV)

15) Which of the following statements regarding cataracts is INCORRECT?

    A. Long-term steroid therapy typically causes an anterior subcapsular cataracts

    B. Hypocalcaemia can be associated with cataracts

    C. Patients can be treated with phacoemulsification

    D. Galactosaemia is the most common metabolic cause of congenital cataracts

    E. Cataracts causes a myopic shift in vision

16) Visual field testing in a patient in the ophthalmology clinic reveals a left-sided contralateral homonymous hemianopia.

Where in the visual pathway is the lesion located?

    A. Left optic nerve

    B. Right optic nerve

    C. Left optic tract

    D. Right optic tract

    E. Optic chiasm

17) A 32-year old male is reviewed in the ophthalmology clinic. Standard automated perimetry reveals a significant visual field defect.

The patient is known to have epilepsy but unfortunately cannot recall his usual anti-epileptic medications.

Which of the following anticonvulsants is the MOST likely culprit?

    A. Topiramate

    B. Tiagabine

    C. Sodium Valproate

    D. Phenytoin

    E. Vigabatrin

18) A 34-year old obese woman sees her GP. She complains of a 4-month history of headache and intermittent transient episodes of 'dimming' or loss of vision, often precipitated by bending over or standing up.

On examination, she has a BMI of 32 and fundoscopy shows bilateral papilloedema.

What is the most likely diagnosis?

A. Amaurosis fugax
B. Migraine
C. Idiopathic intracranial hypertension
D. Cluster headache
E. Brain tumour

19) All of the following extraoccular muscles are innervated by the third cranial nerve except for?

A. Superior rectus
B. Medial rectus
C. Inferior oblique
D. Superior oblique
E. Inferior rectus

20) A 43-year old male presents to his GP after his family noticed that his right pupil was bigger than the left.

On examination, the right pupil fails to constrict in response to light. Furthermore, there is delayed constriction during near vision and delayed dilatation on subsequent focus to distant vision.

Neurological examination reveals absent ankle jerks bilaterally.

What is the MOST likely diagnosis?

A. Argyll-Robertson syndrome
B. Holmes-Adie syndrome
C. Foster-Kennedy syndrome
D. Horner's syndrome
E. Parinaud's syndrome

Ophthalmology Answers

1) E: Topical Tropicamide

This is a typical presentation of acute angle closure glaucoma, an ophthalmological emergency requiring prompt recognition and management. Under normal circumstances, aqueous humour produced by the ciliary body drains to the posterior chamber, through the pupil into the anterior chamber, and finally into the episcleral veins via the trabecular meshwork and Schlemm's canal. In acute angle closure glaucoma, pupillary block, due to the iris adhering to the surface of the lens, prevents drainage of aqueous humour from the posterior into the anterior chamber of the eye. As aqueous humour continues to be synthesized from the ciliary body, the periphery of the iris becomes pushed anteriorly and obstructs the trabecular meshwork drainage system. This causes intra-occular pressure to rise and thus acute angle closure glaucoma. It is one of the causes of the acutely painful red eye.

Visual acuity drastically reduces as a consequence of corneal oedema and patients often characteristically complain of seeing haloes around objects.

Treatment involves the administration of IV followed by oral acetazolamide and topical beta blockers, which collectively work to reduce the synthesis of aqueous humour.

Pilocarpine is a muscarinic agonist, which is also used in treatment, works by constricting the pupil and opening up the trabecular meshwork (as the peripheral iris is no longer bunched up). Tropicamide is a muscarinic antagonist and, by dilating the pupil, it can exacerbate the condition and is thus not a recognized treatment. Topical steroids may be used to reduce the inflammatory response, although frequent long-term use can counterproductively raise intra-occular pressure.

After the acute phase has settled, patients should be considered for laser iridotomies of both eyes to prevent further recurrences.

Khaw PT, Shah P and Elkington AR. ABC of Eyes, Glaucoma-1: Diagnosis. British Medical Journal. 2004;328: 97-9

Khaw PT, Shah P and Elkington AR. ABC of Eyes, Glaucoma-2: Treatment. British Medical Journal. 2004;328: 156-8.

2) D: AV nipping

Primary open angle glaucoma (so-called because unlike in closed angle glaucoma, the irido-corneal angle is open) is an optic neuropathy with characteristic symptoms and signs, the chief risk factor of which is raised intraoccular pressure (IOP). Note that open angle glaucoma is not defined by a raised IOP, as patients with this condition can have normal pressures (of 10-21 mmHg).

Typical signs at fundoscopy include:

1) Optic disc cupping (vertical cup-to-disc ratio of 0.6 or more)
2) Cup-to-disc asymmetry (difference of at least 0.2 between both eyes)
3) Thinning and notching of the neuroretinal rim
4) Vessel bayonetting
5) Peripapillary atrophy
6) Flame shaped disc haemorrhages

Patients with open angle glaucoma are often picked up as a consequence of routine screening by optometrists. In later stages of the disease, patients develop stereotypical visual field defects including arcuate or centro-caecal scotomas, and significant peripheral visual field loss, which can eventually result in tunnel vision.

Management first involves lowering intra-occular pressures using one or a combination of:

a)   *Topical beta blockers (e.g. timolol)*
b)   *Topical alpha 2 agonists (e.g. brimonidine)*
c)   *Carbonic anhydrase (CA) inhibitors (e.g brinzolamide)*
d)   *Prostaglandin analogues (e.g. bimatoprost)*
e)   *Cholinergic agonists (e.g. pilocarpine)*

Topical beta blockers, alpha 2 agonists and CA inhibitors all work by reducing secretion of aqueous humour, prostaglandin analogues work by increasing uveoscleral outflow and cholinergic agonists increase outflow via the trabecular meshwork route. Cases refractory to medical therapy can be treated using laser therapy (e.g. argon laser trabeculoplasty) or surgically (usually trabeculectomies).

Adatia FA and Damji KF. Chronic open-angle glaucoma. Canadian Family Physician. 2005; 51:1229-37

Kwon YH, Fingert JH, Kuehn MH and Alward WLM. Primary Open-Angle Glaucoma. The New England Journal of Medicine. 2009;360: 1113-24

3) C: Grade 3

This grading system is the Keith-Wagener-Barker classification.

1) *Grade 1* = generalised arteriolar constriction manifesting as copper and silver wiring and increased vessel tortuosities
2) *Grade 2* = Arterio-venous (AV) nipping, which represent irregularly located venous constrictions as the hardened arterioles cross their counterpart venous vessels
3) *Grade 3* = cotton wool spots (manifestations of retinal ischaemia and infarction), hard exudates and flame-shaped haemorrhages
4) *Grade 4* = Papilloedema

Note that clinical features of a certain graded hypertensive retinopathy may also have features of a lower grade. There is no grade 5.

Wong TY and Mitchell P. Hypertensive Retinopathy. The New England Journal of Medicine. 2004;351: 2310-7

4) A: Central retinal artery occlusion

This is a classical presentation of central retinal artery occlusion. A branch retinal artery occlusion is unlikely to produce such a profound visual deficit. Patients are often over 60 years of age and may have a history of risk factors including hypertension, ischaemic heart disease, carotid artery disease and diabetes. The pathophysiology involves an embolus lodging into the central retinal artery and severely depriving the retina of its blood supply. The retina thus appears pale, but the so-called 'cherry red spot,' at the fovea, is seen because this is where the retina is at its thinnest, acting as a window to the underlying vascular choroid whose perfusion remains intact. A significant relative afferent pupillary defect (RAPD) delineated by the swinging flash light test (see neurology chapter) is positive in central retinal artery occlusion.

Management in the acute stage involves lying the patient flat, occular massage and IV acetazolamide. Occular massage performed by the patient with the eyes closed for about 15 to 30 mins has the effect of reducing intraoccular pressure (IOP) and dilating the retinal arteries, which collectively help to increase retinal perfusion pressure; additionally, it aids the dislodging of the thrombus/embolus. Specialist ophthalmological intervention may involve anterior paracentesis, which involves needle aspiration of aqueous humour of the anterior chamber to help further lower IOP. Selective intra-arterial fibrinolytic therapy using a microcatheter to cannulate the ophthalmic artery and inject urokinase or t-PA is another option, but not frequently employed due to the need for specialist neuroradiological intervention and the risk of serious complications, namely cerebrovascular accident.

Although central retinal vein occlusion often presents with similar symptoms, fundoscopy findings couldn't appear more different to retinal artery occlusion. In central retinal vein occlusion, there are extensive haemorrhages throughout the fundus, cotton-wool spots, dilated tortous veins, macular and optic disc oedema, collectively producing a so-called 'blood and thunder appearance.'

Beatty S and Eong KG Au. Acute occlusion of the retinal arteries: current concepts and recent advances in diagnosis and management. Journal of Accident & Emergency Medicine. 2000;17: 324-9.

5) B: Non-arteritic anterior ischaemic optic neuropathy

Sudden onset painless unilateral visual loss, most commonly shortly after awakening, is the typical mode of presentation of non-arteritic anterior ischaemic optic neuropathy (NAAION). It is most common in those aged 50 and over, and its pathophysiology involves the infarction of the retrolaminar portion of the optic nerve head supplied by the short posterior ciliary arteries (branches of the ophthalmic artery). Clinical signs include a profound loss of visual acuity, dyschromatopsia, visual field defect, most commonly inferior altitudinal, a segmental optic disc swelling (though may be diffuse) and flame shaped haemorrhages. Patients with abnormally small optic cup-to-disc ratios (less than or equal to 0.2) are at high risk of developing the condition; around 97% of patients with NAAION have such abnormally small cup-to-disc ratios.

Arteritic anterior ischaemic optic neuropathy (AAION) is associated with temporal arteritis. Such patients usually present with headache, scalp tenderness and jaw claudication and are almost exclusively over the age of 60. Additionally, the optic cup-to-disc ratio of the fellow eye is normal. This condition requires urgent and prompt administration of high dose steroids if vision is to be salvaged.

In posterior ischaemic optic neuropathy, which can also present with sudden onset painless visual loss, patients typically develop a central visual field defect. Furthermore, as the more posterior portion of the optic nerve is affected, a normal optic disc and fundus is seen in the acute stages. However, as with anterior ischaemic optic neuropathy, after 6-8 weeks, the optic disc becomes pale due to progressive optic atrophy.

In optic neuritis, there is a unilateral, subacute painful loss of vision, often exacerbated by eye movements. It is the first presenting feature in 15-20% of patients with multiple sclerosis (MS) and occurs in around 50% of patients some time during the course of MS. Patients typically have central scotomas, dyschromatopsia and reduced contrast sensitivity. In two thirds of cases, the fundus appears unremarkable in the acute phase as there is isolated retrobulbar involvement. However, in the remaining third, the optic disc appears swollen due to diffuse papillitis. Over time, optic atrophy occurs causing the disc to become pale.

Kerr NM, Chew S SSL and Danesh-Meyer HV. Non-arteritic anterior ischaemic optic neuropathy: A review and update. Journal of Clinical Neuroscience. 2009;16: 994-1000.

Hayreh SS. Posterior ischaemic optic neuropathy: clinical features, pathogenesis, and management. Eye. 2004;18: 1188-1206.

Balcer LJ. Optic Neuritis. The New England Journal of Medicine. 2006; 354:1273-80.

6) E: Vitreous haemorrhage

Marcus Gunn pupil refers to a relative afferent pupillary defect and is elicited using the swinging flashlight test. Options a) to d) all compromise the rate of neural conduction along the optic nerve. Swinging a pen torch from the unaffected to the affected eye produces an apparent dilation of the pupil as the direct reflex produces a weaker constricting response compared with the intact consensual reflex.

Pearce J. The Marcus Gunn pupil. Journal of Neurology, Neurosurgery & Psychiatry. 1996;61: 520

7) D: Ranibizumab

Age-related Macular Degeneration (AMD) is the commonest cause of irreversible blindness in patients aged 50 or over in the Western world. It has traditionally been divided into dry or wet AMD. Dry AMD is characterised by the deposition of extracellular material between the retinal pigmented epithelium and the underlying Bruch's membrane, resulting in the formation of drusen. Wet AMD, however, is characterised by the formation of a friable subretinal choroidal neovascular membrane. Although wet AMD only accounts for about 10-15% of AMD cases, it more aggressively affects vision and is indeed responsible for up to 80% of cases of registered blindness from AMD. AMD patients typically develop a gradual progressive loss of central vision with relative sparing of the peripheral visual fields. Examination often reveals a central scotoma and metamorphopsia (straight lines appear wavy); the latter occurs because subretinal haemorrhages and drusen disrupt the natural retinal topography. Loss of vision may progress anywhere between over several years (in dry AMD) or more rapidly in wet AMD, particularly if the friable neovascular membranes bleed. Ranibizumab is a monoclonal antibody that targets vascular endothelial growth factor (anti-VEGF). It is administered as a monthly intra-vitreal injection and is used to help slow down the progression of wet AMD.

Chakravarthy U, Evans J and Rosenfeld PJ. Age related macular degeneration. British Medical journal. 2010;340:c981

Jager RD, Mieler WF and Miller JW. Age-Related Macular Degeneration. The New England Journal of Medicine. 2008;358: 2606-17

8) C: Herpes simplex virus (HSV)

Dendritic ulcers are classically associated with herpes simplex keratitis (HSV type 1). Treatment involves acyclovir 3% eye ointment five times daily for at least 3 days after the ulcer has healed. Steroids are contraindicated as they can turn a dendritic ulcer into a more profound ameboid or geographic ulcer.

9) E: Marfan's syndrome

This patient has Retinitis Pigmentosa (RP), an inherited condition characterised by bony spicular pigment deposition in the retina, night blindness (nyctalopia) and gradually progressive tunnel vision (though central visual loss may also occur).

Usher syndrome is the most common systemic association with RP occurring in nearly 30% of patients, and comprises the inherited combination of RP with hearing loss. The typical ophthalmological manifestation of Marfan's syndrome is upward lens dislocation.

Sharma YR, Reddy PRR and Singh DV. Retinitis Pigmentosa and Allied Disorders. JK Science. 2004;6: 115-20.

10) B: Bacterial conjunctivitis

The history and the presence of a purulent discharge strongly supports a diagnosis of acute bacterial conjunctivitis, and makes viral and allergic conjunctivitis less likely. The absence of asthma, hay fever, eczema or any suspicious allergens in the history also makes allergic conjunctivitis less likely. Viral conjunctivitis is typically associated with a mild watery discharge and concurrent upper respiratory tract symptoms such as cough, runny nose and nasal congestion. Bacterial conjunctivitis is most commonly caused by Staphylococcus Aureus and Haemophilus Influenza in adults, and by Haemophilus Influenza and Streptococcus Pneumoniae in children. Contact lens wearers are particularly susceptible to Pseudomonas Aeruginosa, which tends to cause a more severe infection and must be treated aggressively.

Although more than 70% of cases of bacterial conjunctivitis resolve spontaneously within 8 days, treatment with topical antibiotic eye drops can lead to a faster clinical recovery, microbiological cure and also reduces the risk of complications. Topical antibiotics that may be used include chloramphenicol, gentamicin or fusidic acid. Pseudomonas conjunctivitis should be treated with Levofloxacin eye drops. One eye drop should be applied to each eye every 2 hours initially, but applied less frequently as the infection is controlled. As a general rule of thumb, topical antibiotic eye drops should be continued for 48 hours after the infection has resolved.

Patients with Gonococcal conjunctivitis tend to present with copious purulent discharge, which may be associated with genitourinary symptoms. Treatment involves systemic antibiotic therapy (1g ceftriaxone loading dose intramuscularly followed by a course of erythromycin or a tetracycline). Chlamydial conjunctivitis can be treated with a one-off 1g dose of azithromycin or a 1-week course of doxycycline.

Tarabishy AB and Jeng BH. Bacterial conjuctivitis: A review for internists. Cleveland Clinic Journal of Medicine. 2008;75: 507-12.

11) A: Retinal detachment

This history is typical of retinal detachment in an individual at risk (myopia). Three different types of retinal detachment are known:

1) Rhegmatogenous - commonest cause of retinal detachment induced by a full thickness tear or hole in the retina. Fluid from the vitreous cavity enters the potential subretinal space and perpetuates detachment of the retina.
2) Tractional - retinal detachment secondary to contraction of pathological fibrous material on the retina, which may originally be caused by proliferative diabetic retinopathy and trauma.
3) Exudative - secretion of excess fluid into the subretinal space as a consequence of inflammatory conditions or tumours can drive retinal detachment.

Retinal detachment is invariably associated with posterior vitreous detachment. As the vitreous detaches, it tugs on the retina, which aberrantly stimulates the photoreceptors causing photopsia. Further vitreous detachment causes floaters because the vitreous material casts shadows on the retina. However, until the retina itself detaches, vision is not lost, explaining why option B is incorrect. As retinal detachment occurs, there is a loss of visual field, perceived as if a curtain sweeps across the patient's vision. Involvement of the macula leads to a deterioration in visual acuity.

Treatment of retinal detachment includes scleral buckling, pneumatic retinopexy or vitrectomy.

D'Amico DJ. Primary Retinal Detachment. The New England Journal of Medicine. 2008;359:2346-54

12) E: Rheumatoid arthritis

The presentation is that of acute anterior uveitis (also called iritis or iridocyclitis). The pupil is irregularly shaped because the inflamed iris adheres to the cornea (resulting in anterior synechiae) and/ or the lens (resulting in posterior synechiae); anterior uveitis thus also predisposes patients to acute angle closure glaucoma. Anterior uveitis is associated with the seronegative spondyloarthropathies. Rheumatoid arthritis is characteristically associated with scleritis, which presents as an acute red eye with a severe, deep, boring-type pain. Such patients are at risk of scleral perforation. Scleritis contrasts with episcleritis, the latter presenting with much milder pain and representing a far more benign self-limiting condition.

Khan AA, Kelly RJ and Carrim ZI. Acute Anterior Uveitis. British Medical Journal. 2009;339: b2986.

13) C: Vitreous haemorrhage

Diabetic retinopathy is one of the major microvascular complications of diabetes and is the commonest cause of blindness in people aged 30 to 69 years. It can be classified into background, pre-proliferative, proliferative retinopathy and maculopathy.

Prolonged duration of diabetes and poor control of BMs are the two biggest risk factors governing the progression and severity of diabetic retinopathy. Hyperglycaemia stimulates an increase in average retinal blood flow resulting in the formation of microaneurysms, dot and blot haemorrhages and leakage of lipid rich material into the extravascular space, forming hard exudates. This constellation of findings represent background diabetic retinopathy.

Progression of the disease occurs as a result of retinal ischaemia owing to occlusion of capillaries, which can cause retinal infarction manifesting as so-called 'cotton wool spots.' This, along with venous beading and IRMA constitutes pre-proliferative retinopathy. As the retinal ischaemia becomes protracted, patients develop a proliferative retinopathy. This involves the proliferation of new retinal blood vessels under the influence of increased synthesis of vascular endothelial growth factor (VEGF), which triggers neo-angiogenesis. These new vessels that form at the disc or elsewhere (NVD and NVE, respectively) are friable and liable to bleed, which can potentially cause vitreous or pre-retinal haemorrhages. Proliferative retinopathy is further associated with pre-retinal fibrosis. As the fibrous tissue contracts, it can cause a tractional retinal detachment.

If the disease process affects the macula (e.g. hard exudates, haemorrhages etc), then the patient is said to have developed a maculopathy. Background retinopathy is asymptomatic. However, the occurrence of vitreous, pre-retinal haemorrhages, retinal detachment or maculopathy can herald potentially severe and sudden loss of vision.

Watkins PJ. ABC of diabetes: Retinopathy. British Medical Journal. 2003; 326: 924-26

Shotliff K and Duncan G. Diabetic retinopathy: summary of grading and management criteria. Practical Diabetes International. 2006; 23: 418-20

Antonetti DA, Klein R and Gardner TW. Diabetic Retinopathy. The New England Journal of Medicine. 316;13: 1227-39

14) D: Retinitis secondary to Cytomegalovirus (CMV)

This patient has CMV retinitis, which predominantly occurs in immunocompromised hosts. Patients with Acquired Immunodeficiency Syndrome (AIDS) are at high risk, especially if their CD4 counts are less than 50 cells/mm^3. CMV retinitis is the most common ophthalmological complication of AIDS and prior to the advent of Highly Active Anti-retroviral Therapy (HAART), affected up to 40-50% of patients with HIV. Its incidence and related complications has now declined in the developed world, but remains an ongoing problem of developing countries.

Patients present with acute to subacute loss of vision affecting visual acuity and/or visual fields. In the classic form of CMV retinitis, fundoscopic examination shows the characteristic 'pizza pie' or 'cottage cheese with ketchup' sign. Such appearances arise as a consequence of confluent retinal necrosis with patches of haemorrhage. The lesions have usually well-demarcated edges that can advance fairly rapidly over a period of several weeks if left untreated. Treatment involves anti-CMV therapy such as Ganciclovir and the optimization of the patient's HAART regimen. Two other forms of CMV retinitis are recognized. One causing a granular lesion in the peripheries of the retina, which tends to present indolently. The third less common presentation is the frosted branch angiitis.

Banker AS. Posterior segment manifestations of human immunodeficiency virus/acquired immune deficiency syndrome. Indian Journal of Ophthalmology. 2008;56: 377-83

15) A: Long-term steroid therapy typically causes an anterior subcapsular cataracts

The pathophysiology of cataracts is a progressive reduction in lens transparency that occurs because of structural changes to the lens microarchitecture and the accumulation of yellow-brown pigment within the lens. As the lens thickens, there is increased refractory power and thus a myopic shift.

Patients commonly develop gradual and progressive deterioration of visual acuity, reduced contrast sensitivity, colour intensity and problems with glare. Three main types of cataracts are recognised: nuclear sclerosis, cortical and posterior subcapsular cataracts (which patients on long term steroids are at particular risk from).

Although age-related degenerative changes of the lens (i.e. senile cataracts) is the most common cause, multiple systemic associations are recognised as causing cataracts. These include diabetes, corticosteroid therapy, galactosaemia, hypocalcaemia and myotonic dystrophy.

Treatment includes phacoemulsification, intra- and extracapsular cataract extraction. Intracapsular extraction, which involves removing the lens along with the capsule, is now rarely performed in the developed world.

Allen D and Vasavada A. Cataract and surgery for cataract. British Medical Journal. 2006;333: 128-32

16) D: Right optic tract

A lesion of the right and left optic tracts produce a left and right contralateral homonymous hemianopia, respectively. Lesions of the optic chiasm produce a bitemporal hemianopia, typically due to a pituitary tumour. Lesions of the optic nerve produce monocular visual field defects on the ipsilateral side.

17) E: Vigabatrin

Visual field defects are a well recognised adverse effect of Vigabatrin and occurs in 25-50% of adults taking this drug. Due to such a high frequency, adult patients on vigabatrin are routinely screened at 6-monthly intervals for any deterioration in vision. The most common visual field defect is initially a bilateral nasal defect, which can progress to bilateral concentric field defects with relative sparing of central vision. The time of onset from starting the drug to the development of visual field defects can vary from one month to several years.

Ethambutol, an antituberculous agent, is another drug that can commonly cause an optic neuropathy, but instead manifests most frequently as a central scotoma.

Willmore LJ, Abelson MB, Ben-Menachem E, Pellock JM and Shields WD. Vigabatrin: 2008 update. Epilepsia. 2009; 50: 163-73

18) C: Idiopathic intracranial hypertension

Although the patient presents with symptoms and signs of raised intracranial pressure, the history is classically suggestive of idiopathic intracranial hypertension (IIH) instead of a brain tumour. This was previously called benign intracranial hypertension, but the finding that it can lead to blindness in 10% of patients and some form of visual loss in the majority of patients, makes this diagnosis far from benign.

Patients are most often female (ranges from 4:1 to 15:1 female to male ratio) and obese. To fulfill the diagnosis of IIH, there must be no evidence of mass, structural, vascular lesion or hydrocephalus and no other potential cause for the intracranial hypertension.

Common visual field defects seen in patients with IIH include enlargement of the blind spot, loss of the nasal visual fields (nasal step) and generalised constriction of the visual field. Visual acuity may also be affected. Patients can also develop a VIth nerve palsy (false localising sign) manifesting as a horizontal diplopia.

Management initially involves conservative measures, particularly weight loss (which can reduce the progression of papilloedema) and the diuretic acetazolamide. In more refractory cases, surgery including the insertion of ventriculo-peritoneal or lumbo-peritoneal shunts (for diverting cerebrospinal fluid from the ventricles or lumbar subarachnoid space, respectively, into the peritoneal space) and optic-nerve-sheath fenestration for protection of the optic nerve head from the high CSF pressures.

Ball AK and Clarke CE. Idiopathic Intracranial Hypertension. The Lancet Neurology. 2006;5: 433-42.

19) D: Superior oblique

The superior oblique muscle is innervated by the IVth cranial nerve, which is responsible for pulling the eyeball down and out from the neutral position. However, in the adducted position, contraction of the superior oblique pulls the eye inferiorly. Thus, patients with lesions of the IVth cranial nerve typically develop diplopia when going down the stairs as this requires sustaining both eyes in the inferior and adducted positions. The lateral rectus is innervated by cranial nerve VI (abducens), which is responsible for abducting the eye. All the other extraoccular muscles are innervated by the cranial nerve III (occulomotor nerve). A lesion of cranial nerve III causes the eye to move down and outwards due to the unopposed actions of the superior oblique and lateral rectus muscles. Other clinical features of a third nerve palsy include ipsilateral ptosis and pupillary dilation. However, a pupil sparing third nerve palsy can occur in conditions such as diabetes or hypertension where there is microvascular damage to the third nerve. The peripherally located pupillomotor fibers of the third nerve are relatively spared from ischaemic damage but not from causes of extrinsic compression such as tumours or posterior communicating artery aneurysms.

Drake RL, Vogl W and Mitchell AWM. Gray's Anatomy for Students. Elsevier.

20) B: Holmes-Adie syndrome

Holmes-Adie pupil is thought to arise as a consequence of progressive degeneration of the parasympathetic post-ganglionic neurones arising from the ciliary body, which participate in the light reflex. Patients typically develop a tonically dilated pupil that shows no immediate pupillary constriction in response to light. This is combined with an impaired accommodation reflex because there is a delayed constriction response to near vision and a further delayed dilatation in response to switching to distant vision. Note that although there is no immediate constriction in response to light, there is often a slow constriction, after a 5-10 mins exposure to bright light, accompanied by a further delayed dilatation of 15-30 mins in a dark room. The combination of Holmes-Adie pupil and absent deep tendon reflexes is called Holmes-Adie syndrome.

In Argyll-Robertson pupil, the affected pupil constricts during the accommodation reflex but not during the light reflex (i.e. light-near dissociation, similar to Holmes-Adie pupil). In contrast to Holmes-Adie, the affected pupil in Argyll-Robertson syndrome is miotic. The condition was notoriously caused by syphilis and is thought to arise as a consequence of damage to the pre-tectal neurons, which form central connections in the light, but not the accommodation, reflex.

Horner's syndrome is when there is a relatively constricted pupil associated with ipsilateral partial ptosis and anhydrosis. It occurs secondary to a lesion in the sympathetic chain.

Foster-Kennedy syndrome is the constellation of papilloedema in one eye and optic atrophy in the contralateral eye often secondary to frontal lobe tumours.

Parinaud's syndrome refers to the combination, of a selective up-gaze palsy, convergence-retraction nystagmus, light-near dissociation and Collier's sign (eyelid retraction). It is a dorsal midbrain syndrome that can occur due to pineal tumours and almost anything else that compromises dorsal midbrain structures (e.g. infarction).

Martinelli P. Holmes-Adie Syndrome. The Lancet. 2000;356: 1760-1

Pastora-Salvador N and Peralta-Calvo J. Foster-Kennedy syndrome: papilledema in one eye with optic atrophy in the other eye. Canadian Medical Association Journal. 2011; 183: 2135.